S0-ADW-526

THE CRUNCH FITNESS GUIDES

ROAD WARRIOR WORKOUT

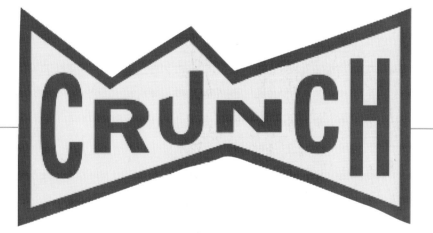

CRUNCH

HATHERLEIGH

NEW YORK

GetFitNow.com Books
An Independent Imprint of Hatherleigh Press

Copyright © 1999 by Crunch Fitness

All rights reserved. No part of this book may be reproduced in any form or by any means, electronic or mechanical, including photocopying, recording, or by any information storage or retrieval system, without permission in writing from the publisher.

GetFitNow.com Books
An Independent Imprint of Hatherleigh Press
an affiliate of W.W. Norton & Company
500 Fifth Avenue
New York, NY 10110
1-800-367-2550
www.getfitnow.com

Before beginning any strenuous exercise program consult your physician. The author and publisher of this book and workout disclaim any liability, personal or professional, resulting from the misapplication of any of the training procedures described in this publication.

All GetFitNow.com books are available for bulk purchase, special promotions, and premiums. For more information, please contact the manager of our Special Sales department at 1-800-367-2550.

Library of Congress Cataloging in-Publication Data

Crunch Fitness,
    The road warrior workout / Crunch.
        p.   cm.   —   (The Crunch Fitness Series)
    ISBN 1-57826-025-6 (alk. paper)
    1. Travel—Health aspects. 2. Exercise. 3. Crunch. I. Crunch. II. Series.
    RA788.5.R57   1999
    613.7'1—dc21   99-35794
                                                                                              CIP

Series Editor: Heather Ogilvie
Cover design: Lisa Fyfe
Text design and composition: John Reinhardt Book Design
Photographs: Peter Field Peck with Canon® cameras and lenses on Fuji® print and slide film

Printed in Canada on acid-free paper

10   9   8   7   6   5   4   3   2   1

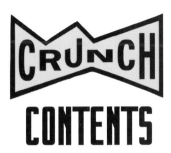

CONTENTS

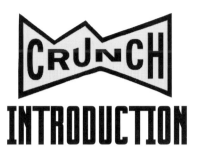

INTRODUCTION

Welcome to CRUNCH! For over a decade, we've been welcoming people of all shapes, sizes, ages, and fitness levels to our gyms. As we've expanded from a tiny, one-room aerobics studio in New York's East Village to cities across the country (and even to Tokyo), we've offered group fitness classes, personal training, and equipment to appeal to everyone from stressed-out workaholics and jet setters to senior citizens and expectant moms. We're living up to our motto, "No Judgements!"

We're aware that some people shy away from joining a gym or from starting a fitness program because they think it demands too great a change in their lifestyle. But at CRUNCH, we believe you shouldn't have to change your lifestyle in order to be fit. In fact, we believe your workout should change to fit your lifestyle. It is our firm belief that the success of a fitness program has nothing to do with how many hours you spend in the gym, but how good you feel when you're outside the gym, living your life.

That's why we've created fitness guides—to show you that no matter what your lifestyle, there's a workout you can do that will complement it and get you fit. For example, we designed the *Road Warrior Workout* for people who spend a lot of time traveling on business. These folks don't have to give up their fitness programs—in fact, by doing a workout specially adapted to life on the road, they can maintain their fitness level and become less susceptible to all the common aches and discomforts of travel.

Get Fit in a CRUNCH is for those people who are trying to shape up in time for a big event—a wedding, a reunion, a trip to the beach. Based on CRUNCH's popular class, Emergency Beach Training, *Get Fit in a CRUNCH* lays out a safe, effective four-week workout, 12-week workout, and six-month workout.

Since the hardest part of any fitness program is starting it, we've written *Beginner's Luck* to help people stay motivated and become more familiar with—and less intimidated by—basic cardiovascular and strength training exercises. It's a workout you can take at your own pace, according to your own goals.

Look for additions to the CRUNCH Fitness Guides targeting time-pressed workaholics, first-time marathon runners, and people who want to eliminate or avoid common back pain and improve posture.

At CRUNCH, we don't want you to conform to some workout fad or a lifestyle of spending more time at the gym than at play. We want to give you workout options that will conform to your lifestyle—without judgement.

Doug Levine
Founder and CEO
Crunch Fitness International, Inc.
www.crunch.com

CRUNCH
ABOUT THE AUTHORS

Dominic dos Remedios designed the Pre-Travel Workout that appears in Part 2: Get Fit to Fly. Currently a personal trainer in CRUNCH's Atlanta gyms, Dominic received a Bachelor of Education, specializing in Human Movement, with honors, at the University of Sydney, Australia. He has coaching certificates in basketball, rugby, and hockey, as well as certification in the following fitness areas: stretch, post-rehab, spin, pre-/postnatal, kickboxing, Posture Perfect, CPR, and first aid. He's also certified by the Australian Council on Health and Physical Education & Recreation, a nationally recognized fitness leaders' course in Australia.

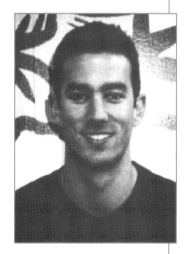

Brian Delmonico designed the stretching routine for the Pre-Travel Workout. A trainer in CRUNCH's 13th Street gym in New York City, Brian began his career as a gymnast at age 6. In his teens, he was on the National Gymnastics Team for three years, and he's a three-time All-American and two-time Big Ten Champion. He graduated from Ohio State University with a Bachelor's Degree in Education and Nutrition. Brian is certified by the USGF in Safety and Stretching—and he has a black belt in Tae Kwon Do.

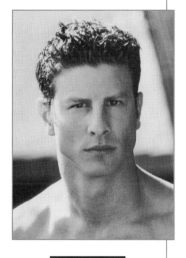

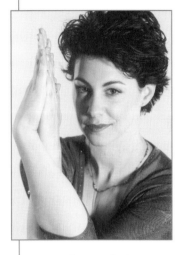

Sara Ivanhoe designed the yoga movements that appear in Part 3: Tranquillity in Transit. Sara teaches at Yoga Works, the premier yoga studio in Los Angeles, where she specializes in rigorous "flow" or "heat" style classes, often called Power Yoga. She studied yoga at the Santa Barbara Yoga Center with Erich Shiffman and attends special workshops with yoga masters from all over the world. Sara has taught the UCLA Women's Gymnastics team and works with seniors, pregnant women, and people with injuries. You can see her leading the yoga workout in the video, "CRUNCH: The Joy of Yoga." She emphasizes enjoying the way the movements feel, without judgment.

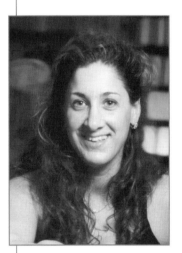

Bonne Marano designed the Hotel Room Workout that appears in Part 4: Check In, Work Out. Bonne is a versatile and exciting instructor with 15 years' experience in the New York area. An AFAA-certified Master Trainer in STEP aerobics, Bonne is a wildly popular instructor at CRUNCH. She has appeared on ABC News (Trainer and the Bride, with Lara Spencer), Good Day New York, and in several fitness videos. She is a regular fitness consultant to *New Woman* and a contributor to *Cosmopolitan, Brides, and Bridal Guide* magazines. Bonne was a featured instructor at *Self Magazine*'s Workout in the Park '97 and '98 and NBC's Health and Fitness Fair '97, and is one of the subjects in a PBS documentary, *Full: Lifestyles of the Formerly Overweight*. She has lectured on Body Image Disorder at symposiums sponsored by Barnard College and has done charity events for MDA and the American Cancer Society.

Stephanie Franklin, MS, RD, CLC, provided the nutrition information in Part 2, Get Fit to Fly. She is a nutritionist in CRUNCH's L.A. gym.

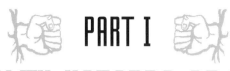

PART I
HEALTH HAZARDS OF THE
FREQUENT FLYER LIFESTYLE

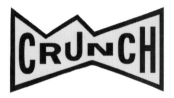

Traveling on business takes you to some of the most exciting places on earth. As a business traveler, you meet new people, explore new cities, and share your talents, products, or ideas with people in foreign cultures.

But eventually the frequent flyer gets fried—both mentally and physically. You may be away from home for a couple days or months at a time. The stress and fatigue of being on the road can hit anytime—after a few days, a few weeks, or before you even board the plane. And even if you don't feel the stress right away, as soon as you start traveling your body is assaulted by health hazards: dry, recirculated air; unhealthy airline "food"; soft, lumpy mattresses; heavy luggage; tiny seats; and dramatic climate changes, to name just a few.

If you're like most road warriors, when you're called to duty to leave on a business trip, your workout is usually the first thing to go. Or maybe you're driven to work out and refuse to give up the muscle tone you've developed. But trying to keep up your regular workout on the road may be inconvenient, unrealistic, and, in some cases, may even do more harm than good.

Consider Jason Smith. A software designer in Los Angeles, for the past several years Jason has worked out four days a week at his local gym. But recently his company promoted him to international VP of sales and sent him out to demonstrate his new software to clients around the globe. In his first month in the new job, Jason was away from home for three weeks. He tried to keep up his intensive workout when he was traveling, but he succeeded only in increasing his frustration: He wasted a lot of time trying to find appropriate facilities. He didn't modify his workouts to account for the considerable energy he had already spent running from appointment to appointment. His eating habits—scheduled around rich business lunches and between flights in airports—left him dehydrated and lethargic. And when he did work out, he felt worse instead of better—his muscles, sore from a late-night workout the evening before, would cramp when he'd find himself stuck in another airline seat the next morning.

Or take Donna Wilson. She was a reporter for a local TV station when she was spotted by a national news producer. He hired her to cover the campaign of a presidential candidate. It was a dream opportunity, but it meant weeks on the road. Donna loved the assignment, but she was under a great deal of stress—not just to produce daily reports from the road, but also to keep in touch with her husband and children at home. She was too stressed to even think about keeping up her exercise program. She lived on caffeine for 18 hours a day, slept poorly, and felt exhausted.

In Jason's case, his regular workout was certainly doing him more harm than good. And in Donna's case, you might think that adding a workout to her schedule would only further exhaust her. But in each case, the right workout—coupled with good eating habits—could improve the traveler's mental and physical well-being.

You may travel for entirely different reasons than Jason's or Donna's. No single profile fits today's road warrior. Who's that sitting next to you on the plane? A salesperson? Model? Executive? Designer? Firefighter? Performer? Missionary? Spy? You all face the same problems:

- Stress: Will you make your connection, your meeting, your show?
- Back pain from carrying luggage and sitting in airline, car, or train seats for hours on end, or from sleeping on poor quality mattresses
- Sore, stiff, or cramped muscles
- Dehydration
- Indigestion from eating foods you're not used to
- Insomnia or poor sleep
- Colds and other "travel bugs" you can easily pick up when your immune system is compromised by dietary and climate changes

THE CRUNCH CURE

Located in cities from New York to Tokyo, CRUNCH gyms are designed for busy people with active lifestyles. CRUNCH caters to people on the go. So our experts are going to tell you how a simple workout that you can do a few days before you travel—and that you can easily modify to suit your current fitness level—can help you reduce the physical and even mental stresses that normally afflict travelers. We'll show you some relaxation techniques and stretches you can do on the plane that will help alleviate common aches and pains—and help mentally calm and refresh you. And once you're in your hotel room, we'll show you a quick, easy workout that you can do right in your room—without special equipment and without incurring the wrath of the neighboring guests.

THE ROAD WARRIOR'S MINDSET

The most important thing to keep in mind during these workouts is your ultimate goal: *To maintain your fitness level and mental well-being.* If you're traveling on business, you're not going away to *improve* your strength or cardiovascular endurance. But if you don't do some sort of exercise, you will actually lose some of the gains, some of the strength and endurance, you've worked so hard for. Experts estimate that after two weeks of no exercise, you will lose 15 percent of your aerobic capacity. And not exercising for four weeks decreases your cardiovascular fitness by 50 percent! While your aerobic fitness level suffers first from a break in your exercise routine, your strength suffers, too. After about six weeks away from the gym, you'll lose the gains you've developed from strength training.

The workouts in this book, therefore, are designed to help you maintain your current fitness level. We'll show you moves that will help boost your energy as well as moves that will help relax you. But these moves are *not* designed to push you. When you're traveling, you want to avoid sore muscles, which may only add to the other aches and stresses associated with travel.

Another important thing to keep in mind is that by using the time you have to yourself—be it on the plane, in an airport, or in a hotel room—to clear your mind and focus on your health and well-being, you will help yourself relieve stress. We'll show you some meditative techniques in Part 3. And the Hotel Room Workout in Part 4 will help your body release endorphins, the hormones that naturally produce feelings of well-being.

The physical aches and pains of traveling are only complicated by

SAY WHAT?

Blocked ears are a common complaint among travelers. You don't have to suffer from chronic ear infections to experience the painful pressure of blocked ears during flights. Ears can even stay blocked long after you land, compromising your hearing. To help "open" your ears:

- Chew gum or yawn during takeoff and landing
- Take a decongestant a half hour before landing
- Hold your nose while trying to blow through it

mental and emotional stress. Even travelers who thrive on meeting new people get lonely on the road. You may miss your spouse, friends, family, or pet. Making a little time for yourself every day to call, write, or even just think about them may help you feel less frazzled.

When you're traveling, of course, time is everything. And one of best aspects of our workouts is that they're brief. You can do them in just 25 to 40 minutes. That gives you more time to finish those last-minute errands before you leave—or take in a few more sights of the city you're visiting.

THE LOWDOWN ON JET LAG

Almost any physical discomfort associated with traveling gets chalked up to jet lag. Here are just a few:

- fatigue
- inability to concentrate
- dehydration
- swelling in legs and feet
- the feeling of being in motion even after you've landed
- diarrhea and constipation
- indigestion
- trouble sleeping at night, and
- trouble staying awake during the day

Many of these symptoms have the same cause: disrupted sleep patterns. As you cross time zones you reset your wristwatch, but your body clock is not so easily adjusted. It is usually easier to recover your normal sleep pattern after flying west, when you gain time, than after

HOW DRY AM I?

You've no doubt heard that the air on board flights is very dry. In fact, the humidity is only about 10 percent—even dry cities like Tucson have higher humidity (around 25 percent). But while you may be aware of the facts, you may not recognize when you are dehydrated, and you may not associate certain discomforts with dehydration. Got a bad headache after landing? Eyes sore? Sluggish? Not digesting your food properly? You're probably dehydrated.

In addition to drinking plenty of water—eight ounces for every hour of flight time, you should moisturize your skin and use natural saline drops to replenish the moisture in your eyes (that's especially important if you wear contacts that can become uncomfortable or pop out if they become too dry). Apply moisturizer when your face and hands are a little damp—that helps lock in the moisture.

flying east, when you lose time. In general, though, experts estimate that for every time zone you cross, you need one day to recover your energy and reestablish your normal sleep/wake pattern. (Sleep/wake patterns are also called "circadian rhythms.") That means if you fly from Los Angeles to New York, crossing three time zones, you could need three days to recover!

Obviously, you can "trick" your circadian rhythms by napping, adjusting your diet, and timing your exercises. Experts, however, often disagree on the benefits of napping on flights. Some say that you should sleep on a flight only if you're traveling while it is night where you are going. But if it is daytime at your destination, you should try to stay awake. The idea is that you want to be able to fall asleep easily at night at your destination. Others think that anytime you can catch a few winks you should. A good rule is to set your watch to the local time of your destination as soon as you board your flight. This will help mentally prepare you and help you decide whether you should nap.

Some frequent travelers advise scheduling flights that will arrive at your destination's evening time. That way, you can simply go to bed when you arrive. Others prefer to book flights that leave in the evening because these flights are often less crowded so there's more room to stretch out. More often than not, though, business travelers don't have much of a choice in scheduling their flights, but if you do, you might want to consider the pros and cons of morning and evening travel.

BAGGAGE AND THE BACK

Time was, travelers packed up their seemingly indestructible Samsonite Touristers, heaved them into the trunk, and prayed they found a skycap available at the airport. Then the luggage industry came up with a major innovation: the wheel. Soon, happy travelers were dragging their 50 pound Touristers around the airport as if they were obedient Labradors.

Another innovation was not far behind. In an effort to save time by breezing by the baggage carousel, business travelers demanded an upgrade of the flight bag: the carry-on. The trouble is, people attempt to pack the same amount of stuff into their carry-ons as they would have packed into their regular-size suitcases. As a result, the carry-ons bulge beyond their FAA-approved dimensions—and beyond their recommended weight limits. Needless to say, they don't fit under the seat in front of you. You are stuck trying to shove them into the overhead compartment—with everyone else's overstuffed carry-on. Once again, modern men and women are heaving luggage over their heads, slinging garment bags over their shoulders, and sacrificing precious leg room for their laptops and dumbbells.

We're not the airline industry. We're not going to tell you how to pack and what to check. But there are a few tips you should keep in mind to avoid sore muscles:

- Use suitcases with built-in wheels and long handles, so you can pull them rather than lift them.
- Avoid bags with shoulder straps that can put a great deal of pressure on your neck, shoulder, and spine.
- Consider using a backpack as a carry-on bag. It distributes weight evenly across your back and leaves your hands free.
- When you do lift luggage, bend your knees and lift with your legs, not with your back.

Adding to the fatigue caused by readjusting to another time zone is the atmosphere on board a plane. The cabin pressure at a plane's cruising altitude is similar to the air pressure in the High Sierras. If you're not used to mountain life, you may suffer from lethargy. Poor circulation will cause swelling in your legs and feet. Therefore, it's important to wear loose, comfortable clothes and shoes, and get up and walk around a few times during the flight. If you've got time in an airport between connecting flights, use it to walk around the terminal.

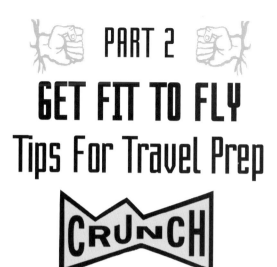

PART 2
GET FIT TO FLY
Tips For Travel Prep

How well you feel during your trip and how well you adjust to the environment at your destination depends in large part on how you prepare yourself physically. And that doesn't just mean what exercises you do—it also means what foods you eat and drink.

In this chapter, we're going to discuss what you can eat before, during, and after a flight to avoid jet lag as well as digestive disorders associated with traveling. We'll also recommend some snacks and supplements you can pack as a Food First Aid Kit and discuss ways to adjust to the local cuisine.

Next, we'll take you through a pre-travel workout that's short enough to fit into your busy schedule in the days before your trip. You'll get a good workout, but you'll avoid being sore and exhausted before you even leave.

EATING ON THE FLY

It's the day before your big trip. You're mind is racing with thoughts about all the work you have to do before you leave, what you're going to pack, and who's going to water the plants—you haven't had time to think about dinner. Maybe you'll just grab a burger at the drive-thru.

Better not. That greasy burger may end up being your traveling companion for the next 24 hours. Whether you're traveling by train, plane, or automobile, it's important to put a little time and effort into maintaining good eating habits before you leave. That's because what you eat before your trip can affect your mood, energy levels, and immune system—not to mention your physical comfort.

So let's start again. You've got a five-hour flight tomorrow morning. What should you eat for dinner tonight?

First, you should try to eat fairly early in the evening, say six or seven o'clock, says L.A.-based CRUNCH nutritionist, Stephanie Franklin. Second, the meal should be well balanced with some protein, carbohydrates, and fat. Eating a high-carbohydrate meal late at night can make you feel sluggish the next morning, especially if you're going on an early-bird flight. In addition, drinking alcohol or caffeine the night before a flight can dehydrate you and keep you from getting a good night of rest.

If you're leaving on an afternoon flight, avoid eating a heavy breakfast or eating high-fat foods likes muffins, danishes, and other pastries. If eating at the airport is your only option, look for cereal with skim milk, yogurt with a whole-grain, low-fat muffin or bagel or try to find an energy bar. Skipping breakfast altogether is definitely not a good idea.

If your flight leaves in the evening, eat regularly throughout the day, without skipping meals, to make sure that you're not ravenous when you get on the plane. If you're hungry, you may be tempted to eat airline food, like those little packets of peanuts. One's not so bad, but if you're hungry and eat a whole bunch, their calories and fat will add up fast.

Another way to resist eating airplane food is to pack a few snacks for the flight. You might consider energy bars, dried fruit, whole-grain crackers and peanut butter, and whole-grain bagels. Steer clear of snacks that have to be refrigerated, such as milk, yogurt, and cheese— if you don't get a chance to eat them within two hours, they could spoil. Also, try to avoid "empty calorie" snacks such as cookies, brownies, and potato chips. These foods provide a lot of fat and calories with little nutritional value.

By all means, take along some bottled water! It is sometimes difficult to be served enough water throughout the flight. Experts recommend drinking 8 ounces for every hour of flight time in order to avoid dehydration. Bear in mind that not all liquids are adequate substitutes for water. Soda is generally not a good substitute for water, because the carbonation can make you feel bloated (gas expands at high altitudes). Coffee, tea, and other caffeinated beverages have a diuretic effect that can further dehydrate you. What's more, relying on caffeine to perk you up in order to counteract the effects of jet lag may backfire—you may be stimulated for a while, then have even more trouble sleeping later or otherwise adjusting to a new time zone. Too much caffeine can actually cause fatigue—and an irregular heartbeat.

It's common knowledge that drinking alcohol on a plane not only dehydrates you more quickly than not drinking anything, it can also give you a bad hangover when you land. That's because alcohol's effects are doubled when you fly. One bloody mary (or beer or glass of wine) in flight has the effect of two bloody marys (or beers or glasses of wine) on the ground.

Although airline food has the same culinary ranking as hospital food, airlines are paying more attention to the health concerns of passengers and are offering healthier items. If you call ahead, you can usually order a vegetarian, low-sodium, or other special meal. First-class and business-class passengers have more options than coach passengers, but more options means it's easier to go overboard, nutritionally speaking. Creamy salad dressings, cheese and cream sauces, fatty meats, rich desserts.... If you indulge in some of these offerings, you're likely to end up with a first-class case of indigestion when you land.

Food First Aid Kit. In addition to antacids and pain relievers, there are some foods, herbs, and nutritional supplements that can help you avoid or relieve common disorders associated with traveling. For instance, if you're prone to motion sickness, you might want to consider taking a supplement of ginger one hour before the flight. If you're anxious or restless, chamomile or valerian root tea can help relax you.

Some herbs and supplements have been touted for their ability to counteract the effects of jet lag, including valerian root, chamomile, kava kava, and passionflower. Foods high in tryptophan, an amino acid, promote sleep, so eating one of the following foods before bedtime may help you drift off more easily: turkey, bananas, figs, dates, yogurt, tuna, whole grain crackers, or nut butter. At bedtime, try to avoid alcohol, caffeine, sugar, tobacco, cheese, chocolate, sauerkraut, bacon, ham, sausage, eggplant, potatoes, spinach, and tomatoes. These foods contain tyramine, which increases the release of norepinephrine, a brain chemical stimulant.

For morning energy, try eating whole-grain cereals and breads along with a source of protein, such as skim or low-fat milk, yogurt, or low-fat cottage cheese. These foods provide you with sustained energy throughout the morning.

CAUTION: Some herbal remedies that claim to give you energy can be harmful. Products that contain Ma Huang (a.k.a. ephedra) can cause serious side effects, such as an irregular heartbeat. Some people can tolerate products containing ephedra without any side effects, but it is wise to talk to your doctor before taking any supplements that could have adverse effects.

There's been a lot of talk recently about melatonin and its ability to combat jet lag. Recent studies have suggested that taking a supplement of melatonin an hour before bedtime will help you fall asleep and "reset" your body clock after traveling across time zones. Melatonin is a hormone your body produces in response to darkness, and it reaches its peak level about 2:00 in the morning. The hormone is found in meats, fruits, vegetables, and grains, so eating certain foods can have the same effect as taking a supplement. However, *people on certain medications or who suffer from certain diseases or are pregnant should not take melatonin.* Again, consult your doctor before taking this supplement for jet lag.

Local Flavor. Your dietary troubles are not over when you land. Now you've got all those rich business lunches to eat, not to mention adjusting to the local cuisine. Here are three important rules:

1. Don't overeat, especially if you're eating late at night.
2. Avoid fried foods.
3. Pack an antacid.

Don't be afraid to ask questions about how a dish is prepared. Most restaurants are willing to honor your request if you ask that a food be prepared a certain way.

If you experience frequent heartburn, avoid fried foods, carbonated beverages, foods with a high fat content, and highly spiced foods. Pack an antacid. Ginger can help relieve symptoms of nausea and indigestion. Parsley, gentian, and chamomile, all of which come in both capsule form or as a tea, can be helpful as well. Peppermint tea can help relieve gas pains.

THE PRE-TRAVEL WORKOUT

As you probably know, for any workout to be complete, it must address the following components—cardiovascular, strength, and flexibility. The Pre-Travel Workout is no exception.

CARDIO TRAINING: Improves the heart and lungs, bringing oxygenated blood to all the working muscles. It also helps burn fat.

STRENGTH TRAINING: Builds strong muscles, which help protect the bones, support the joints, and aids in burning fat.

FLEXIBILITY TRAINING: Stretching improves your range of motion through the joints and reduces the risk of injury.

The following workout incorporates all these components, and it undoubtedly contains many moves you're already familiar with.

We've specially designed it to target all the muscle groups. In your current workout, you may focus on special areas you want to tone, but in the days before you travel, it's important to cover all the muscle groups. That's because you're likely to use muscles during your trip—lifting luggage, dashing to make connections, sitting in awkward positions—that you may not have used in a while. As a result, those unused muscles are more prone to cramps, pulls, and soreness. This workout will give them all a good stretch and exercise them, which will help you avoid such soreness.

Although this workout is complete, it is also conveniently brief. It is designed to be done in a minimum of time (approximately 25 to 40 minutes), which is convenient if you've got a lot of things to do before your trip.

Keep in mind that the workout is designed to maintain your fitness level and not push you too hard—you don't want to get on a plane and be sore from a workout. So while you can modify this workout according to your fitness level (for instance, increasing the weights of the dumbbells or performing more reps), be careful that you're not overdoing it.

The workout spans six days, alternating strength training with stretching. As with any good fitness program, brief aerobic segments should begin and end each day's workout as a warm-up and cooldown. On strength training days (Days 1, 3, and 5), begin with a brief full-body stretch as well. On these days, you can adapt the workout according to your fitness level and personal goals. For instance, you choose the weight of the dumbbells and barbells (3 to 5 lbs), you decide the resting time between exercises (between 15 and 30 seconds), and you can expand the aerobic sections, performing the exercises in a circuit, if your goal leans more toward aerobic fitness than toward strength building.

Finally, while this workout uses equipment you can find in any gym, it incorporates exercises that are easily modified when no gym is available. The Hotel Room Workout, described in Part 4, is a modification of this one, so that when you get on the road, you'll be doing a routine you're already familiar with.

- **Day 1:** Strength training: Push muscles—chest, triceps, abs
- **Day 2:** Stretching
- **Day 3:** Strength training: Pull muscles—back, biceps, abs
- **Day 4:** Stretching
- **Day 5:** Strength training: Shoulders, legs, abs
- **Day 6:** Stretching

We'll go through the Strength Training Days 1, 3, and 5 first, and then we'll demonstrate the stretches for Days 2, 4, and 6. Don't forget to begin each day of the Pre-Travel Workout with 10 to 15 minutes of aerobic activity (treadmill, bike, jumprope, etc.) to get your heart rate up.

DAY 1: PUSH MUSCLES: CHEST, TRICEPS, ABS

Exercise	Reps (or time duration)
Warm-up	10–15 minutes
Bench Press	15
Military Push-ups	15
Dumbbell Flies	15
Knee Raises	15
Incline Bench Press	15
Wide-arm Push-ups	15
Dumbbell Flies on incline bench	15
Knee Raises	15
Dumbbell Bench Press with rotation	15
Dumbbell Incline Bench Press with rotation	15
Jump Rope	4 minutes
Tricep Bench Dips	15
Tricep Extension	15
Crunches	15
Tricep Push-ups	15
Tricep Kickbacks	15
Seated Overhead Tricep Extension	15
Cool-down	5–10 minutes

DAY 1 →

Begin with an aerobic warm-up and full-body stretch. For each of the moves described below, do 15 reps, one time, unless otherwise indicated (you can increase reps according to your fitness level).

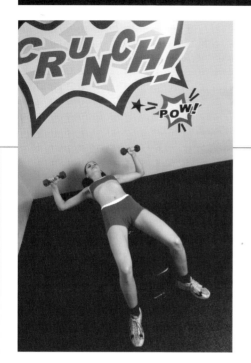

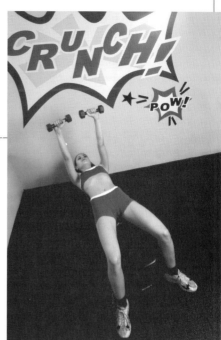

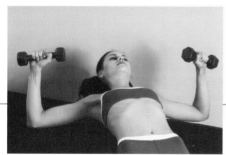

BENCH PRESS

Your chest muscles are the first group of muscles you'll be working, and the first move is the bench press. Lie on your back on the bench. Grasping dumbbells in each hand with palms facing away from you, bend elbows so that they rest just below your back level. Raise dumbbells straight up until your arms are fully extended above you. Bring the dumbbells down again to just above your chest.

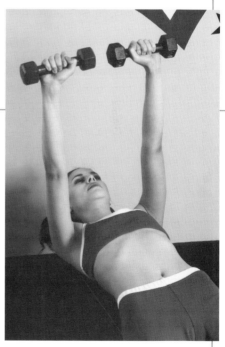

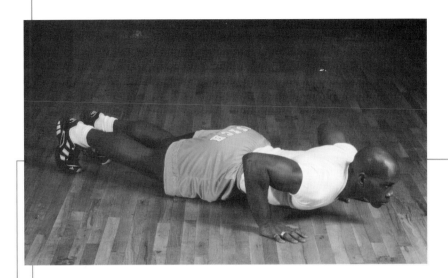

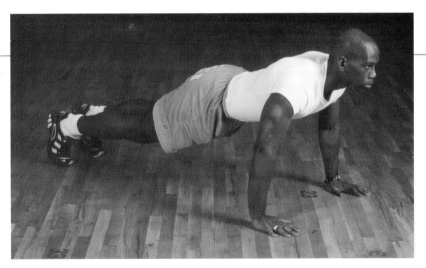

PUSH-UPS

Do this first set of push-ups military-style, with your hands placed directly beneath your shoulders. Make sure you look forward as you do them, not down. While push-ups mainly work the chest muscles, they also work the triceps and abs.

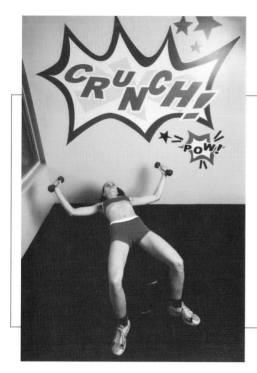

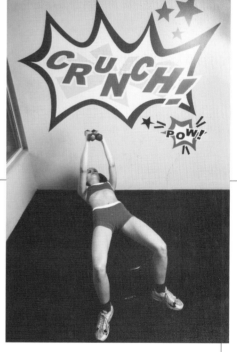

DUMBBELL FLIES

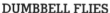

Lie flat on your back on a bench or on the floor, and extend your arms straight out to your sides (if you are using a bench, your elbows should be slightly bent below bench level at the start). Keeping arms straight and hands stationary, bring dumb-bells together over your head so that your palms are facing each other. Squeeze your chest when you bring the dumbbells to the top.

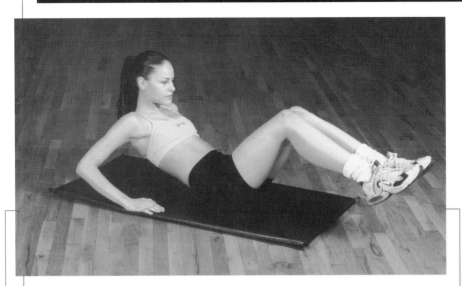

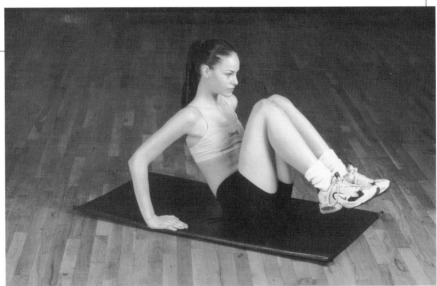

KNEE RAISES

To give your chest muscles a brief rest, work your abs with knee raises. These can be done sitting, lying, or hanging, depending on the desired degree of difficulty. If you're doing them lying on floor, as shown, extend your arms out to the side, but keep your elbows slightly bent. Your legs should be slightly off the ground at the start. Raise your knees to your chest.

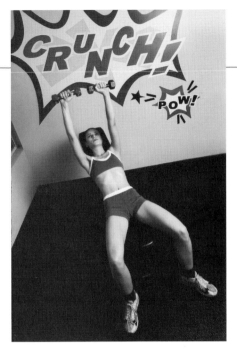 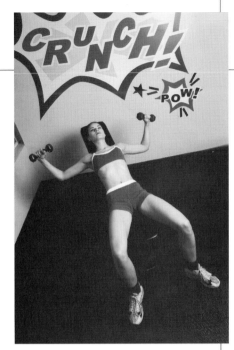

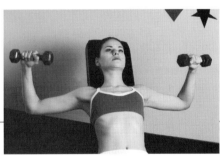

INCLINE BENCH PRESS

Repeat the same bench press as before, only incline the bench to a 45 degree angle. By shifting the angle, the move targets your upper chest muscles.

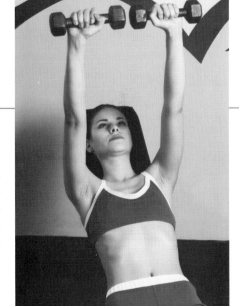

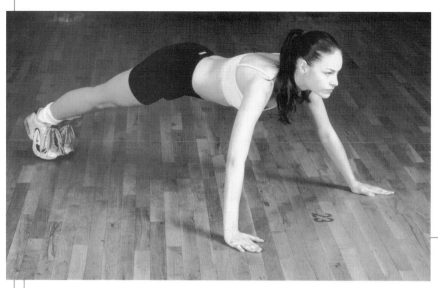

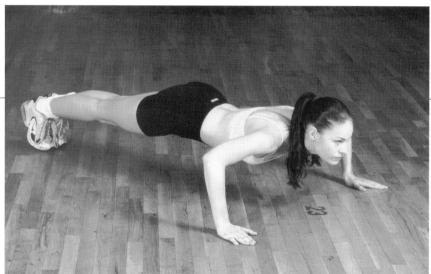

PUSH-UPS

This time, do wide-arm push-ups. Taking the arms wider works the outer chest muscles.

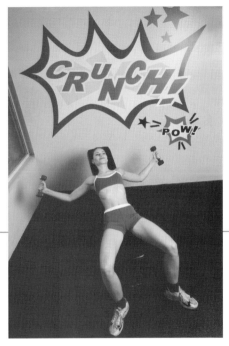

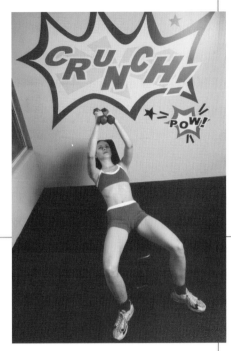

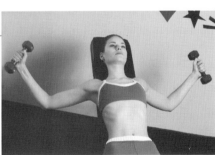

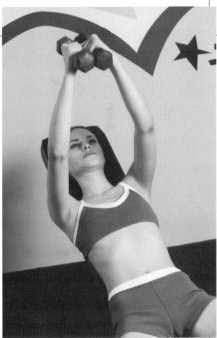

DUMBBELL FLIES
ON INCLINE BENCH

Do the same flies as described earlier, only incline the bench on a 45 degree angle. Like the incline bench press, these flies work the upper chest.

Time to give your chest another break and work those abs. Do another set of knee raises.

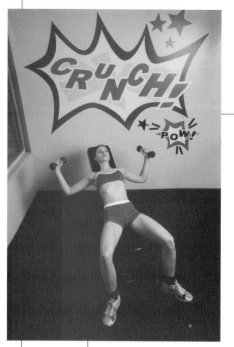
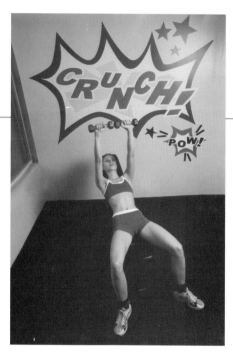

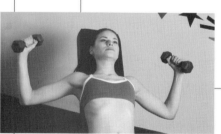

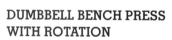

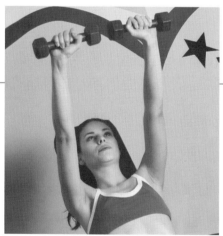

DUMBBELL BENCH PRESS WITH ROTATION

Lying on a horizontal bench, rotate one arm from bench press to flies position. In other words, begin on the exhale, with palms facing together, and as you raise your arms, rotate your palms so that they face outward at the top. Repeat with other arm.

DUMBBELL INCLINE BENCH PRESS WITH ROTATION

Adjust the bench to an incline angle, and perform the same move as above. Once again, simply by switching angles, you're working different areas of the same muscle group.

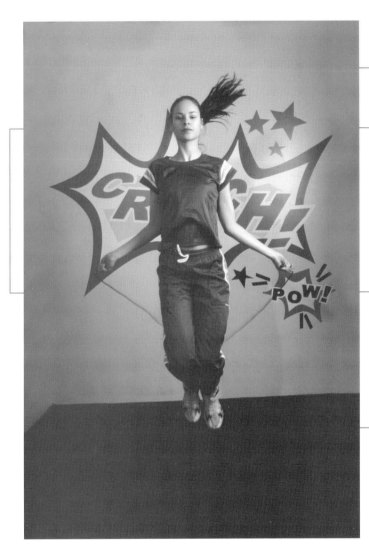

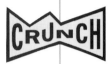

CARDIO BREAK

Stretch out your chest and then jump rope or do step-ups for 4 minutes. Step-ups involve stepping onto and off of a bench (step, or other raised object that can support your weight), alternating legs. The step up should be no higher than your hips.

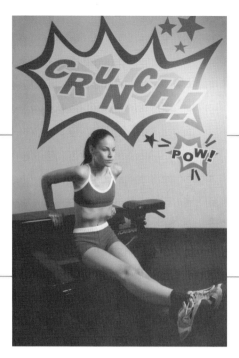

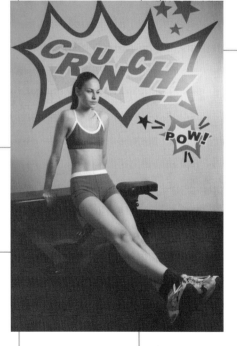

TRICEP BENCH DIPS

Sit on the bench and extend your legs so that your knees are not bent, crossing your legs at the ankles. Hold the end of the bench with your fingertips facing forward and slide your butt off the bench. Lower yourself toward the floor by bending at your elbows. Straighten up your arms again to complete the movement, but don't let your elbows lock. Keep your butt close to the bench.

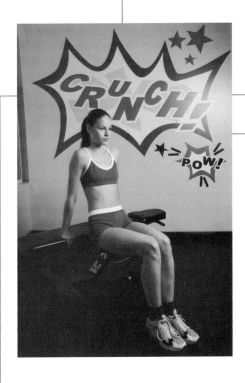

If you want an easier dip, bend your knees.

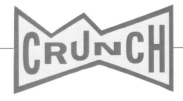

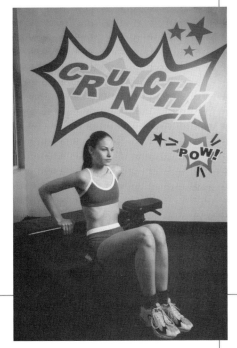

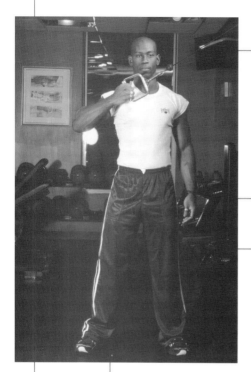

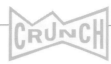

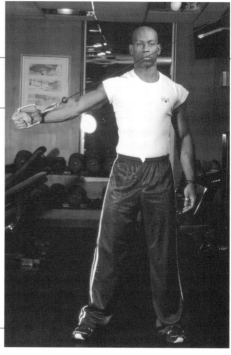

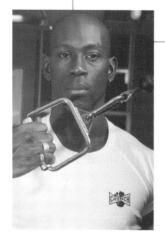

TRICEP EXTENSIONS
(CABLE CROSS-OVER)

With your hand in the "hammer position" (gripping as you would a hammer), grab the cable and pull across your chest and out to the side. Do not lock your elbow. Repeat with other arm.

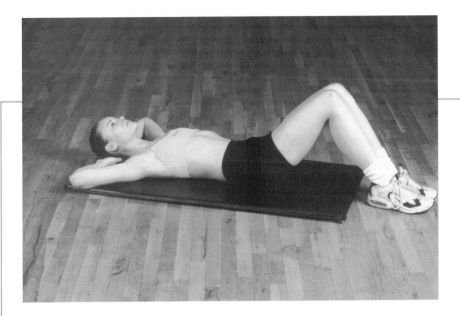

CRUNCHES

Rest your triceps briefly and work those abs again! Be careful not to pull on your neck as you lift your shoulders. For maximum benefit, do not bring your shoulders all the way down to the floor between reps.

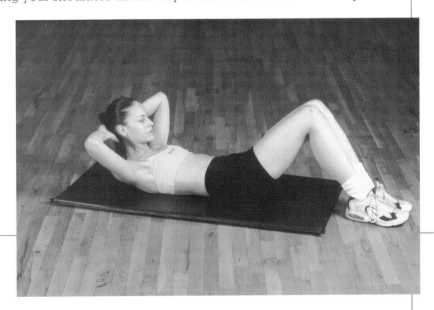

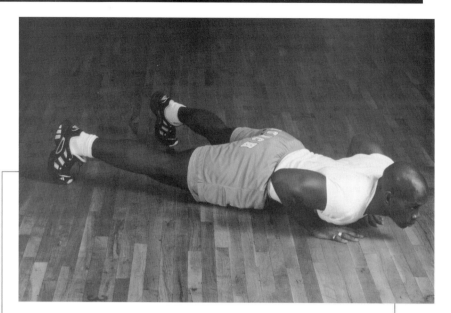

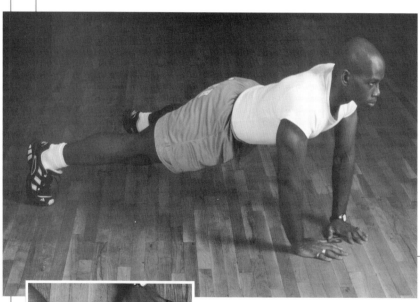

TRICEP PUSH-UPS

For these push-ups, keep your hands to-gether, forming a triangle under your chest. Your legs should be wider than hip-distance apart. This push-up variation is probably the most difficult. It really targets the triceps.

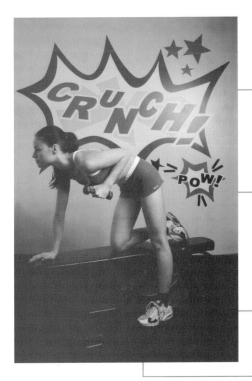

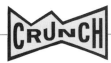

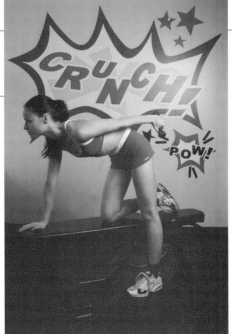

TRICEP KICKBACKS

Kneeling on bench, or standing with one foot a long stride out in front of you, hold a dumbbell in one hand in front of you with your elbow bent. Straighten out your forearm behind you, being careful not to "swing" your arm back. Repeat with the other arm.

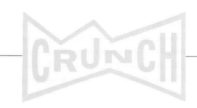

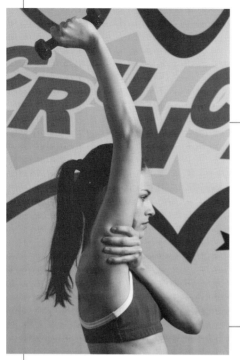

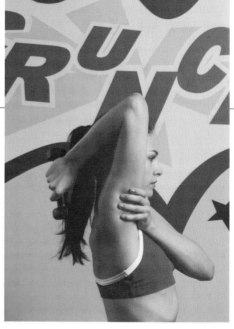

SEATED OVERHEAD TRICEP EXTENSION

Hold a dumbbell in one arm that is fully extended over your head. Bend your elbow back, bringing the dumbbell back behind your head. You can support the arm with your other hand. Repeat with the opposite arm.

COOL DOWN

Jump rope or do step-ups—you're flushing blood through your muscles.

DAY 3: PULL MUSCLES: BACK, BICEPS, ABS

Exercise	Reps (or time duration)	
Warm-up	10–15	minutes
Wide-arm Pull-ups	15	
Wide-grip Lat Pull-downs	15	
U-grip Pull-ups	15	
Lat Pull-downs	15	
Knee Raises	15	
Crunches	20	
Arch-ups	2 sets of 15	
Seated Rows	15	
Seated Back Flies	15	
Crunches	15	
Reverse Crunches	15	
Jump Rope	4	minutes
Barbell Bicep Curls	15	
Barbell 15s	15	
Dumbbell Preacher Curls	15	
Knee Raises	15	
Dumbbell Bicep Curls	15	
Dumbbell Hammer Curls	15	
Dumbbell Concentration Curls	15	
Wrist Raises	15	
Venting	100	
Cool-down	5–10	minutes

DAY 3 ↷

Warm up and stretch out. Do 15 reps of each of the following moves, one time, unless otherwise indicated.

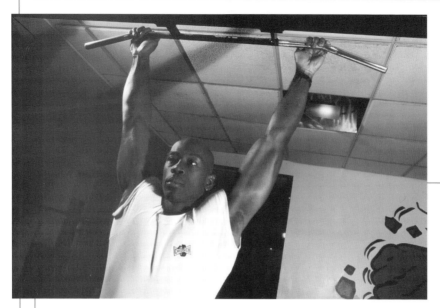

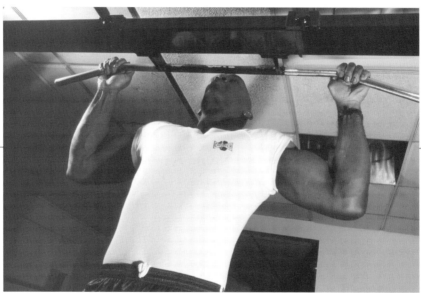

WIDE-ARM PULL-UPS

Today we're going to start with the back muscles, and chin-ups really work your back. For the wide-arm variation, make sure you're using an overgrip and your hands are wider than shoulder-width apart.

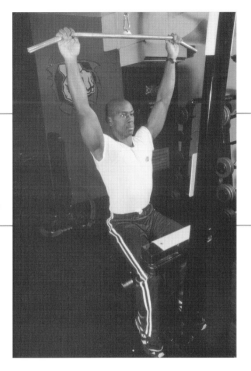

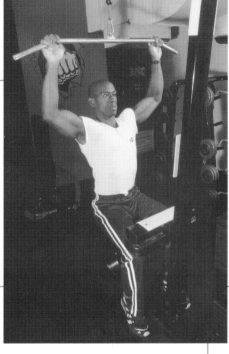

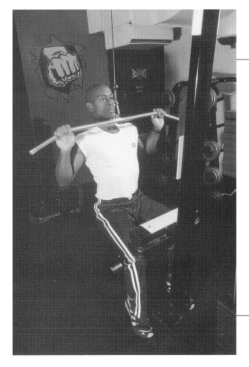

WIDE-GRIP LAT PULL-DOWNS

While sitting, pull the bar down in front of your head. Do *not* pull down in back of your head—that can strain your neck.

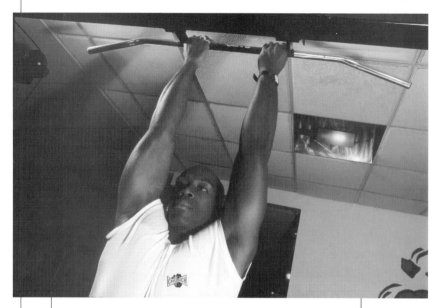

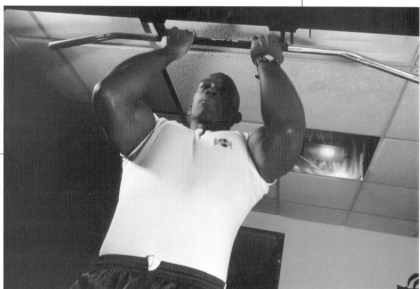

U-GRIP PULL-UPS

Do another set of chin-ups, only this time, use an undergrip and place hands shoulder-width apart.

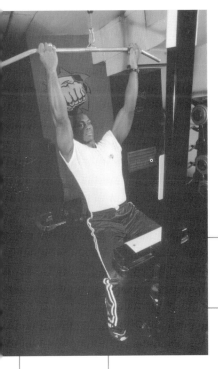

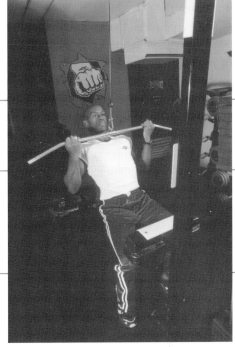

LAT PULL-DOWNS

With a shoulder-width grip, lean back and pull bar to middle of chest. The narrower grip targets different areas of the back than the wide-grip lat pull-downs did.

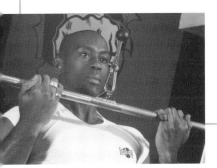

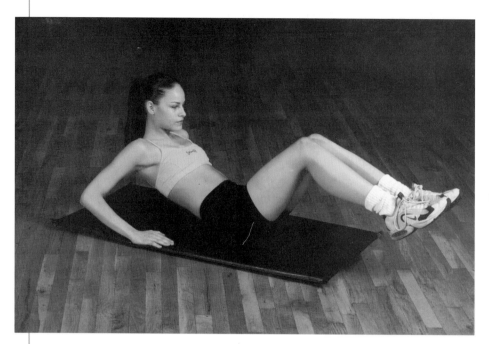

KNEE RAISES

Time to rest your back and work your abs. Today, do 20 reps of knee raises.

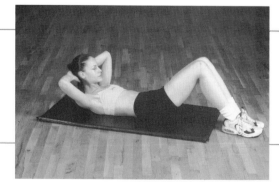

CRUNCHES

Do 20 reps. You heard me.

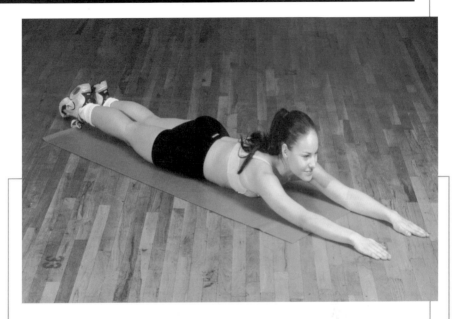

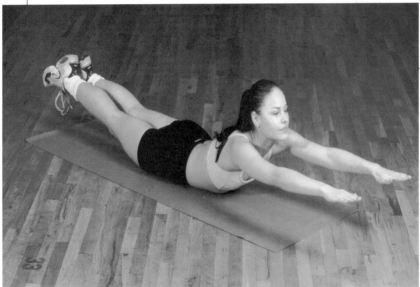

ARCH-UPS IN SUPERMAN POSITION

Lie on your stomach on a mat and keep your knees together. Raise knees and extend arms in front of you. This move is good for the back and butt. Do 2 sets of 15 reps.

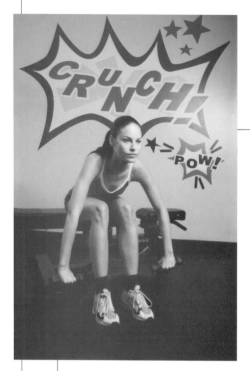

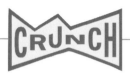

SEATED ROW

Being careful not to round your shoulders and keeping your back straight, sit on the bench and hold dumbbells in each hand below bench level, at your ankles. Keep your elbows bent. Pull dumbbells up to knee height, squeezing shoulder blades at the top. Keep your back flat or you'll place too much stress on it.

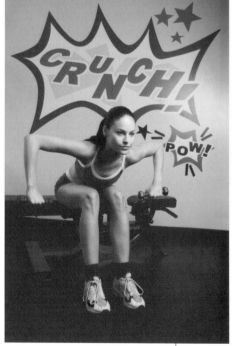

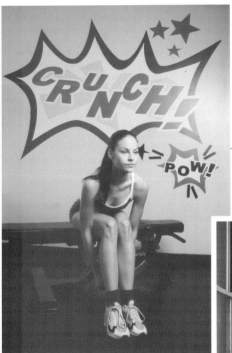

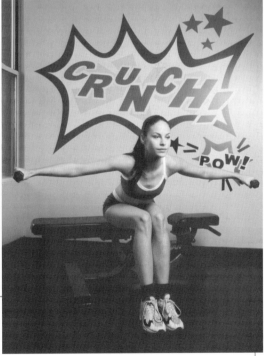

SEATED BACK FLIES

In the same starting position as the Seated Row, extend arms out to sides and up to shoulder height.

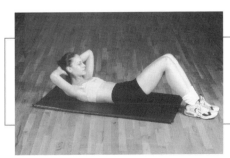

CRUNCHES

Do 15 reps.

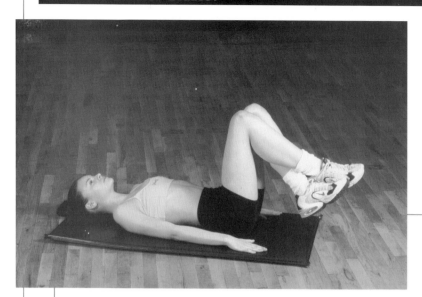

REVERSE CRUNCHES

Lie flat on your back with your arms at your sides. Start with your legs just above the floor, crossed at your ankles. Raise your legs and bring your butt off the ground. Hold the position for a couple seconds, then slowly lower legs. Do 15 reps.

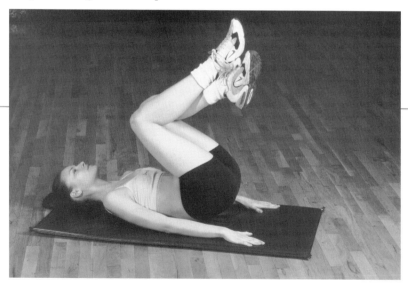

CARDIO BREAK

Jump rope or do step-ups for 4 minutes.

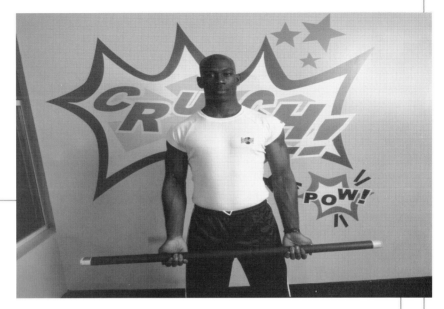

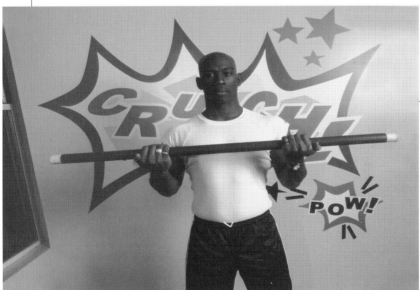

BARBELL BICEP CURLS

Stand straight, and, with an underhand grip, hold barbell down in front of you. Lift barbell to shoulder level and slowly lower down again.

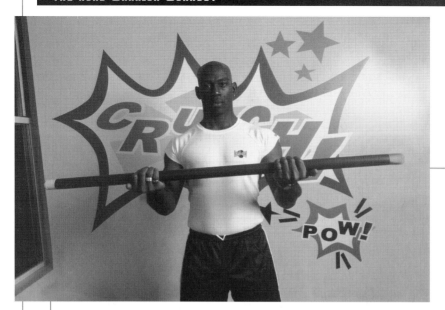

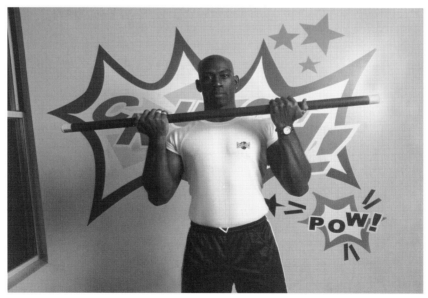

BARBELL 15s

Lift barbell half-way up to chest five times, repeat, then do 5 full curls.

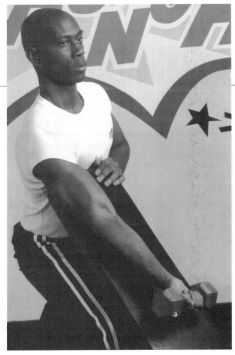

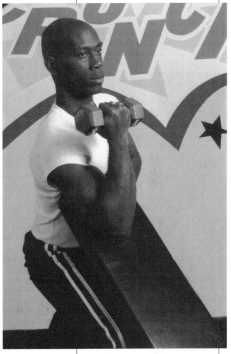

DUMBBELL PREACHER CURLS

While standing, lean over an incline bench and extend one arm down the length of the bench. Bring the dumbbell up to your chest.

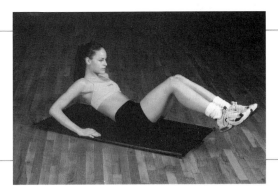

KNEE RAISES

Your biceps can take a brief rest, but your abs can't.

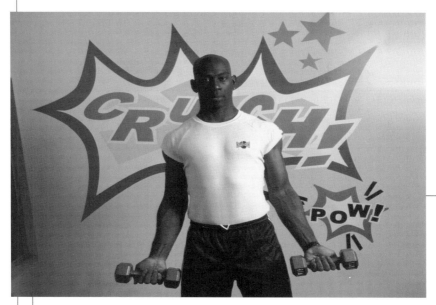

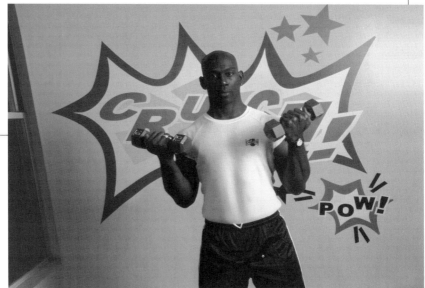

DUMBBELL BICEP CURLS

Hold dumbbells at your sides and curl them up to your chest.

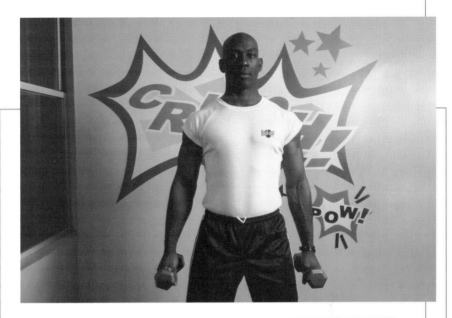

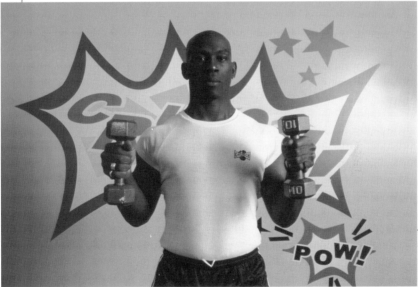

DUMBBELL HAMMER CURLS

These curls are done with your hands in the hammer position. Keep a slight bend in your wrist so you'd see your fist at the top if you were looking in a mirror. You can alternate arms or work both arms together.

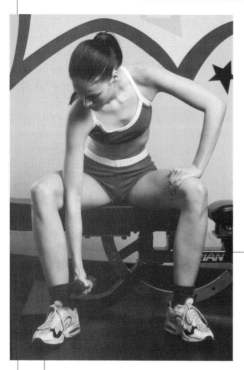

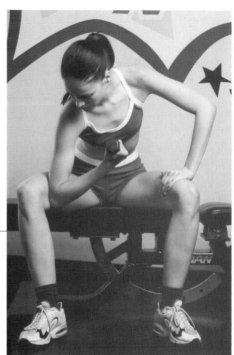

DUMBBELL CONCENTRATION CURLS

Sit on a bench and lean slightly forward, but keep your back straight. With legs slightly apart and one elbow bent at the inside of one knee, curl the dumbbell up to your shoulder and then lower again. You may place your free hand behind your elbow for support and to keep the elbow from moving.

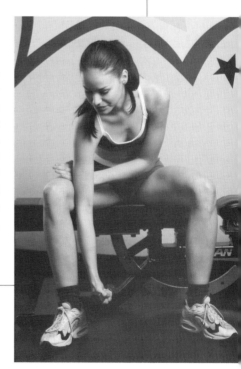

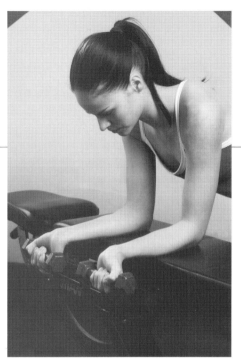

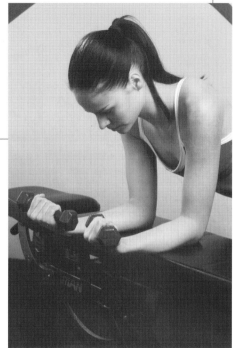

WRIST RAISES

Kneel, with elbows and forearms straight on the bench
and wrists (palms up), clear-
ing the bench. Holding a
dumbbell, raise wrists up
above bench level and
down below bench level.
This move works your forearms.

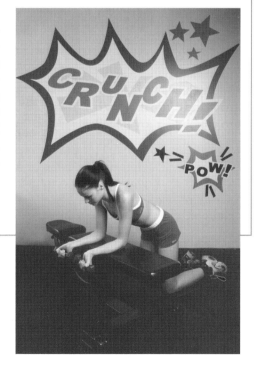

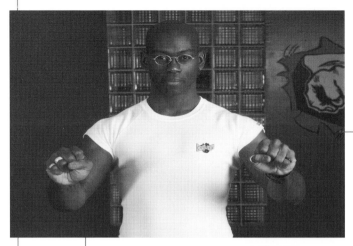

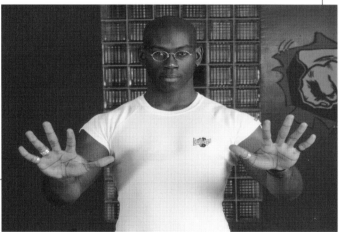

VENTING

Rapidly move fingers from fist position to fully extended wave position. You may think this move looks silly, but it really works the whole forearm. Do 100 reps.

COOL DOWN

Jump rope or do step-ups.

DAY 5: SHOULDERS, LEGS, ABS

Exercise	Reps (or time duration)	
Warm-up	10–15	minutes
Traveling Lunges	15	
Squats	15	
Wall Squats	15	
Crunches	15	
Leg Presses	15	
Crunches	15	
Toe Raises	15	
Calf Raises	15	
Leg Extensions	15	
Hamstring Curls	15	
Crunches	15	
Fire Hydrants	15	
Extended Leg Raises	12	
Butt Raises	20	
Bent Knee Raises	15	
Dumbbell Flies	15	
Upright Rows	15	
Circle Flies	10	
Reverse Circle Flies	10	
*Overhead Push-ups (optional)	10	
Cool-down	5–10	minutes

DAY 5 ↷

Warm up and stretch out. Do 15 reps of each of the following moves, one time, unless otherwise indicated.

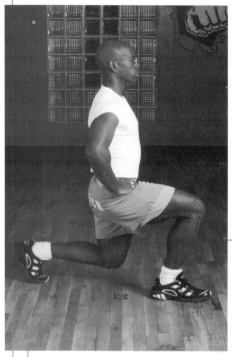

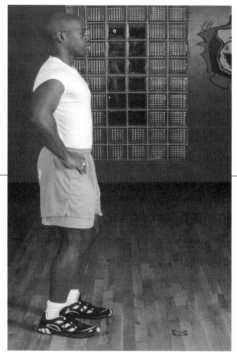

TRAVELING LUNGES

Standing straight up with hands on hips, lunge to full stride with right foot and lower left knee to the ground. Stand up again, moving forward, and lunge with your left foot. Travel forward in this manner for 20 lunges. Holding weights is optional.

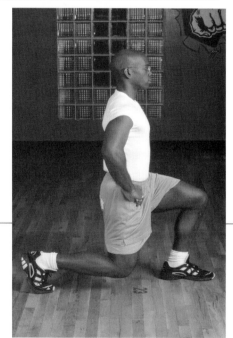

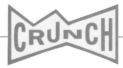

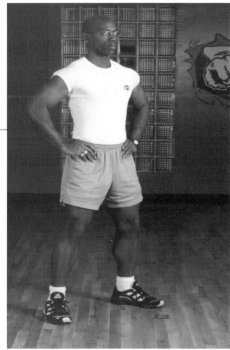

SQUATS

Stand with your feet hip-width apart and your hands on your hips. Squat down directly; don't go forward. You want your thighs to form a 90 degree angle with your calves.

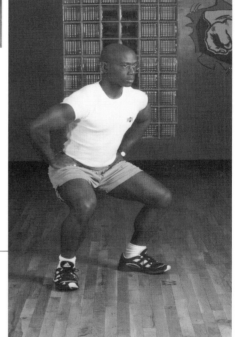

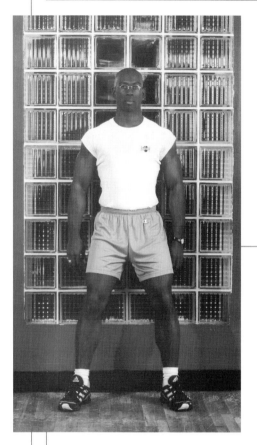

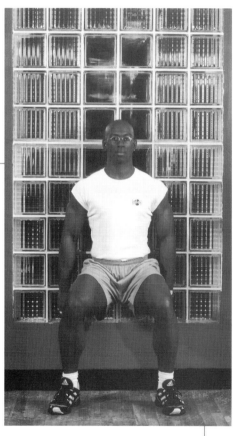

WALL SQUATS

Stand with your back and palms against a wall. Slowly squat down into a sitting position against the wall. Using a stability ball is optional.

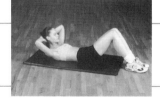

CRUNCHES

Our favorite exercise will be your favorite, too!

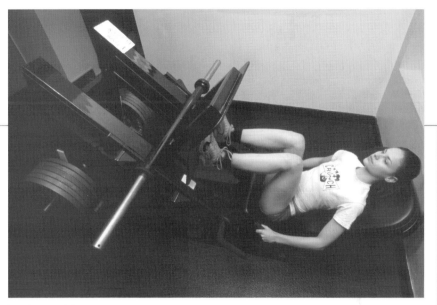

LEG PRESS

Feet may be placed low on the platform or high, shoulder-width apart. Press the weights up until your legs are nearly straight (don't lock your knees).

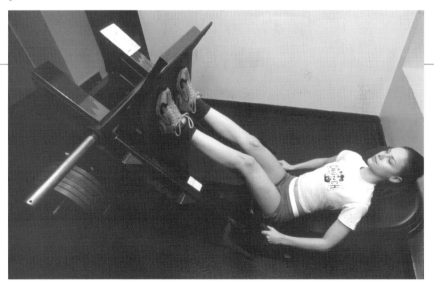

CRUNCHES

You're working your abs a little bit more each day . . .

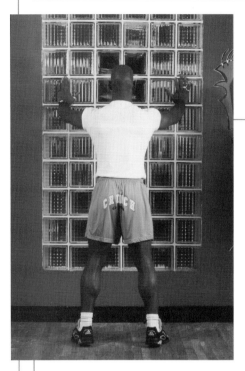

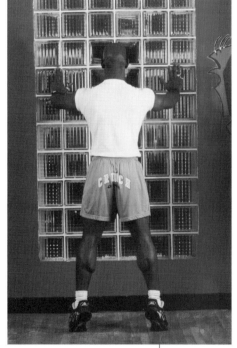

TOE RAISES

Standing with hands against a wall or bar, lift yourself up on your toes and lower yourself back down again.

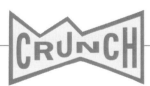

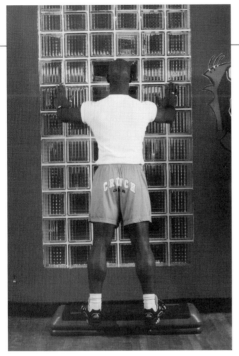

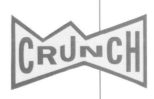

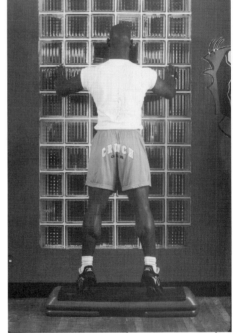

CALF RAISES

Standing on your toes on a step or platform, raise up on your toes and then lower your heels below step level.

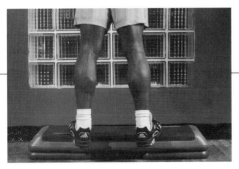

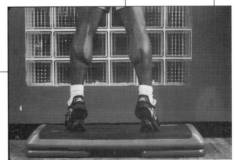

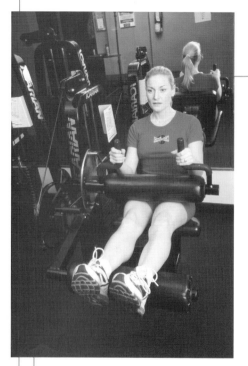

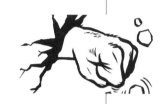

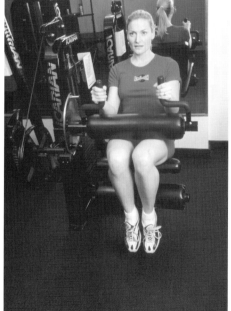

HAMSTRING CURLS

While sitting and grabbing the bars with both hands, lower the weight slowly down to a bottom point of a right angle between the upper leg and lower leg. Flex at the knee, raising the feet until almost completely straight-legged.

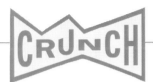

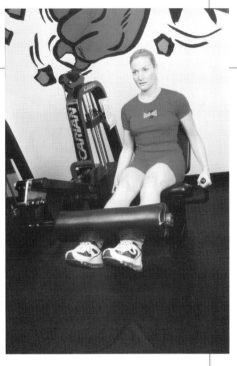

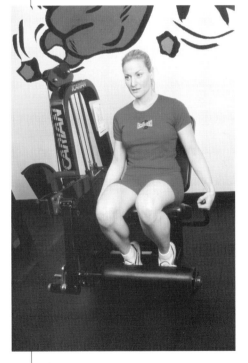

LEG EXTENSIONS

Sitting, holding the bars at your sides and resting the pad on top of your ankles, slowly raise the pad until your legs are fully extended in front of you. Raise the pad up to a right angle between your upper leg and lower leg.

CRUNCHES

It's that time again.

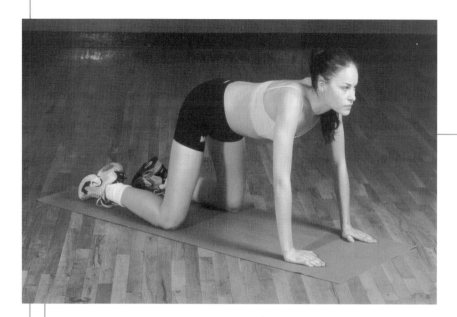

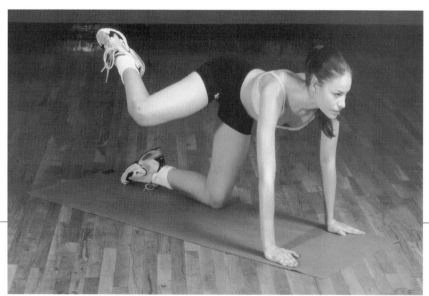

FIRE HYDRANTS

Get on all fours and raise one leg out to the side. Don't tilt your body. Keep your other leg straight, and make sure you have a slight bend in your arms. Repeat on opposite side.

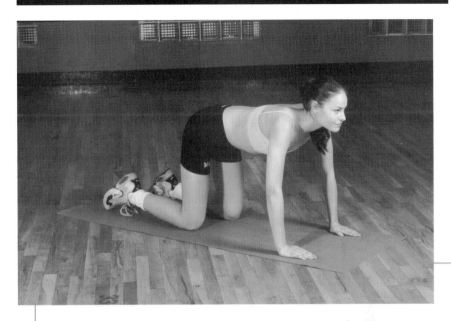

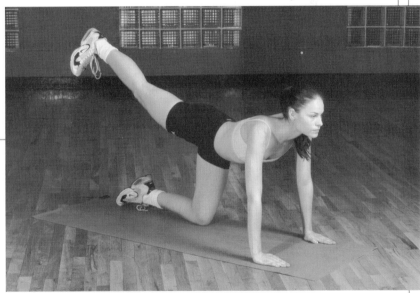

EXTENDED LEG RAISES

Start again on all fours, but this time extend one leg out and back. Your heel should be farther back than your toe. Raise the extended leg up slightly, then lower. Do 12 reps. Repeat with opposite leg.

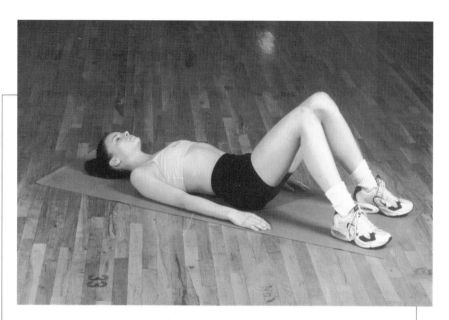

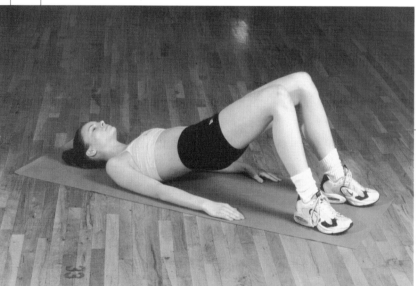

BUTT RAISES

While lying on your back with arms flat your side and knees up, raise your butt. Do 20 reps.

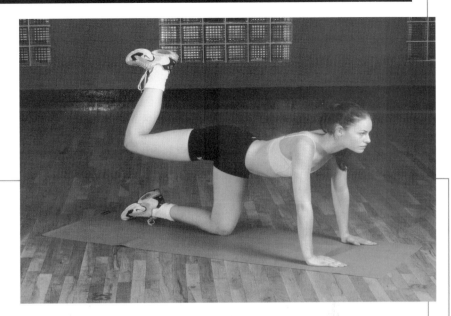

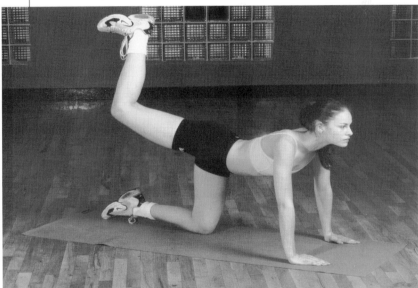

BENT KNEE RAISES

Take the same position as extended leg raisers, but bend the knee. Raise leg up. Don't arch your back! Alternate legs.

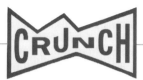

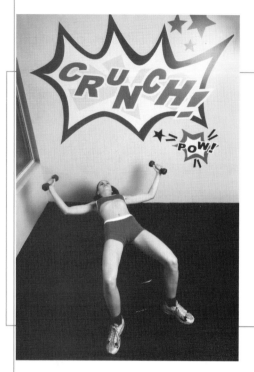

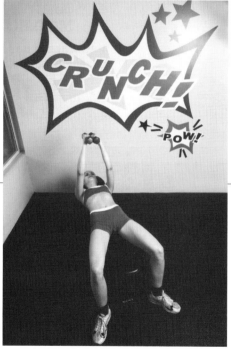

DUMBBELL FLIES

Use 3 lb. dumbbells and face
grips outward. Do 10 reps.

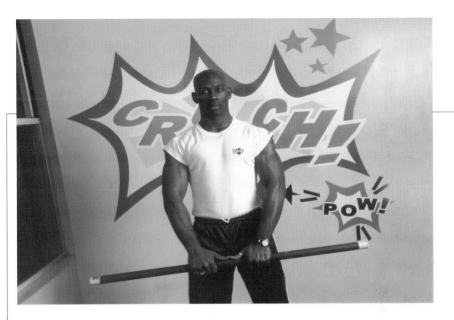

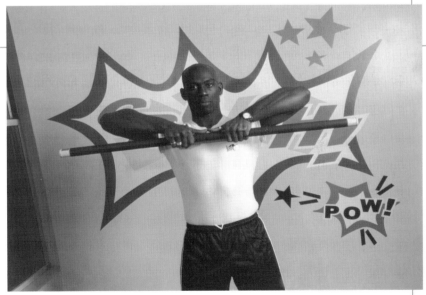

UPRIGHT ROWS

Stand, holding dumbbells (or barbell) with an overgrip at your hips. Bring the weight straight up to your chin, bending your elbows out to the sides.

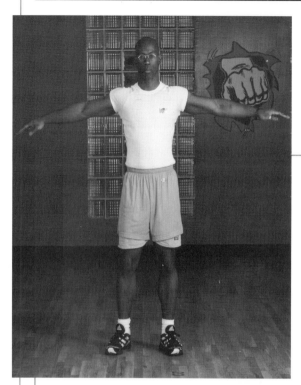

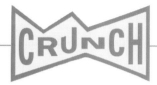

CIRCLE FLIES

You can do these over-head or with arms straight out to your sides. Move arms in small circles. Do 10 reps.

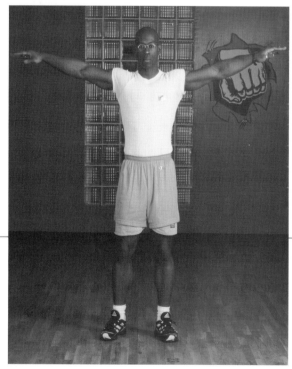

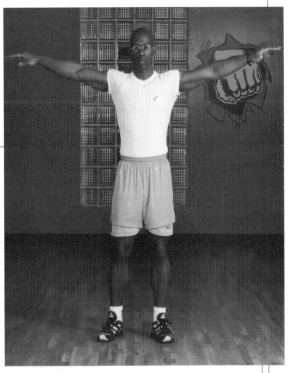

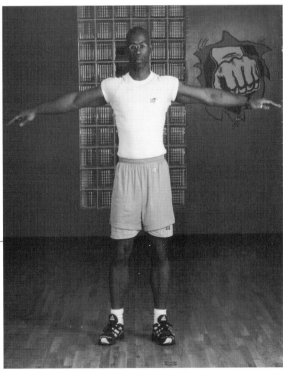

REVERSE CIRCLE FLIES

Change the direction of the circles, for example, from clockwise to counterclockwise. Do 10 reps.

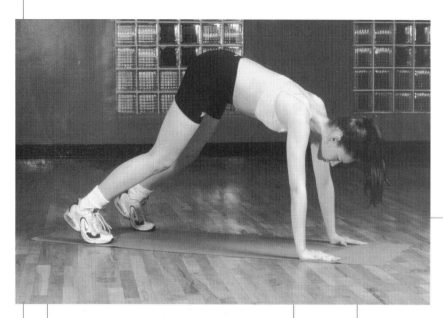

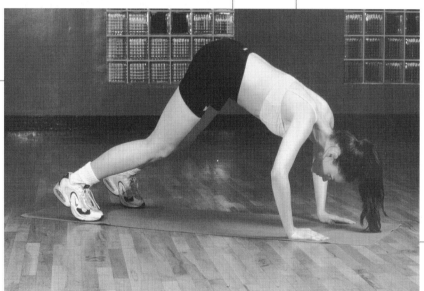

Optional: OVERHEAD PUSH-UPS

With legs slightly bent, feet hip-distance apart, bend over and touch the floor. Hands should be wide apart. From this starting position, bend your elbows and bring your chin down toward the floor. Don't fall on your head!

DAYS 2, 4, AND 6

Hold each position for 15 seconds unless otherwise noted.

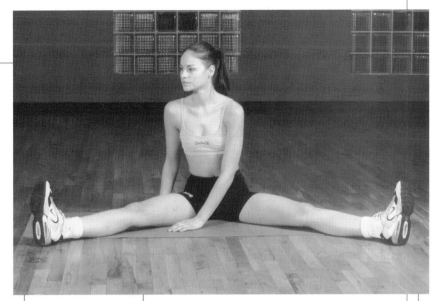

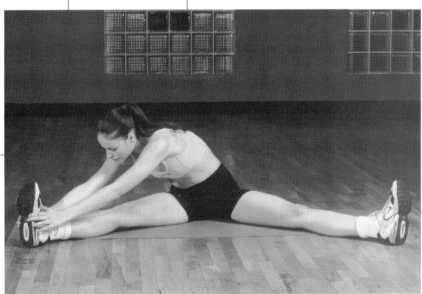

Sitting with legs straight out in a wide straddle, reach down your right side, bringing chest as close to knee as you can. You don't have to be able to touch your feet. Repeat on left side.

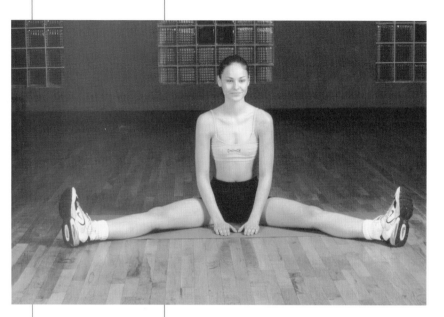

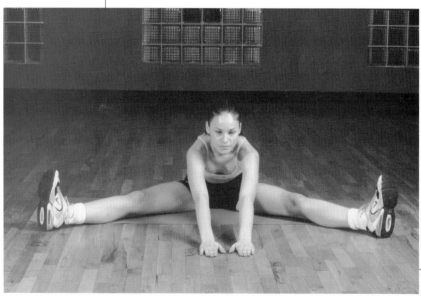

Walk hands up the middle, bringing chest as close to floor between your legs as you can.

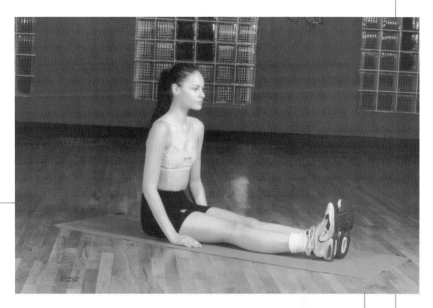

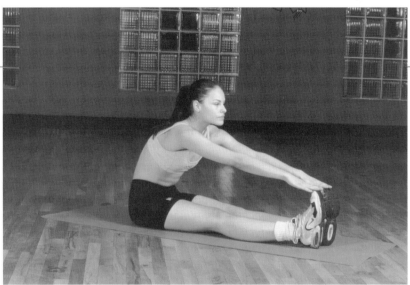

Bring legs together and walk your hands up toward your feet. This is a pike stretch.

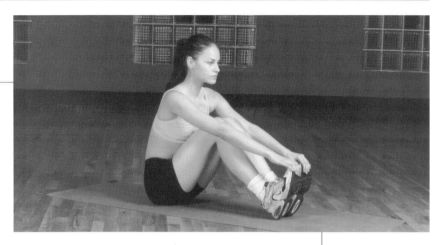

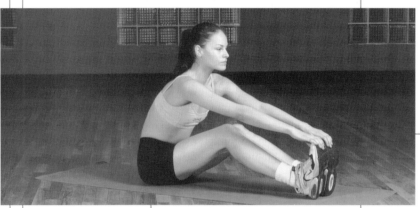

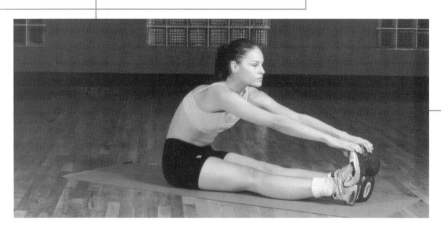

Bring knees up to chest and grab your toes. Straighten legs out as much as you can. Flex your toes and pull back.

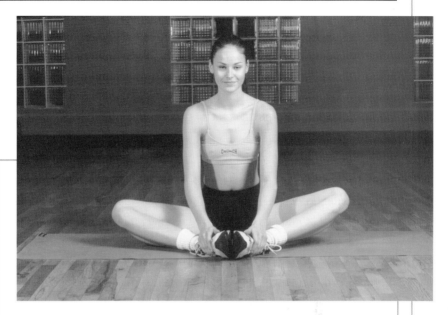

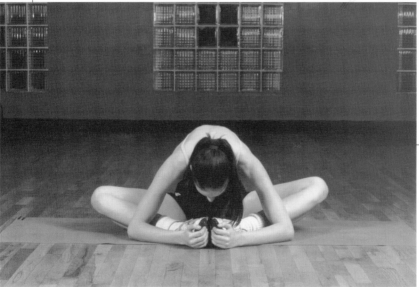

Bring your feet into your middle in a butterfly position. Put your hands on your feet and put your head down.

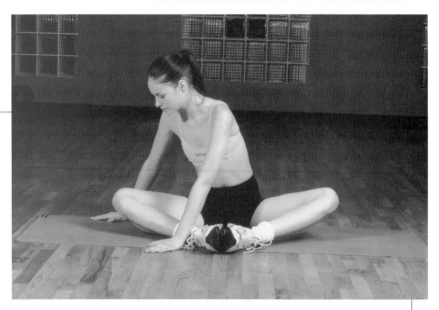

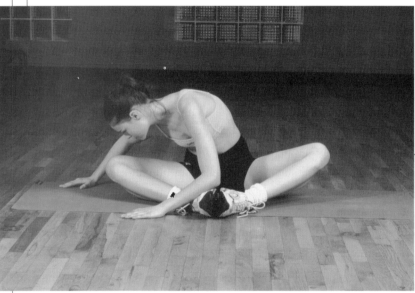

Placing your hands on the floor on either side of your knee, lower your head toward your knee. Repeat on other side.

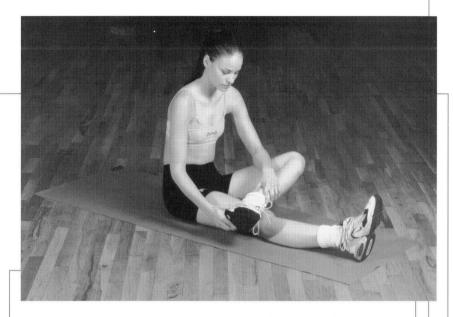

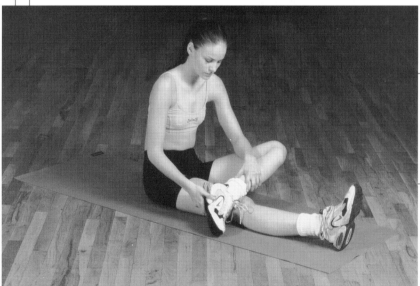

Put one leg out straight and put opposite leg's foot to straight leg's knee. Rotate ankle each way.

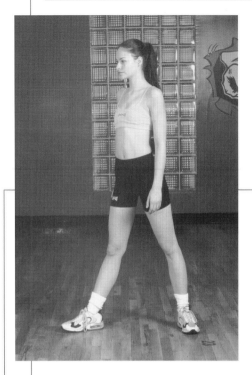
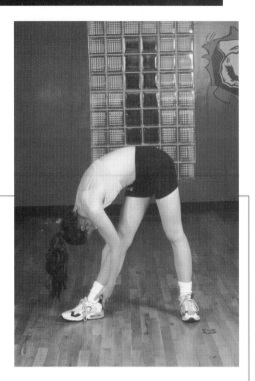

Stand up, with legs apart and feet pointing out. Turn body to the right, making sure your chest is in line with your knee. Work hands down your right side to your feet. Repeat on left side.

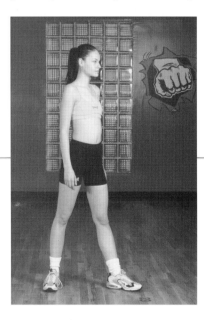
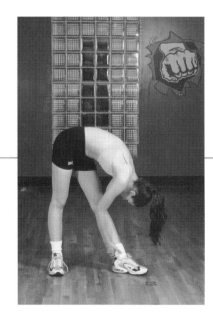

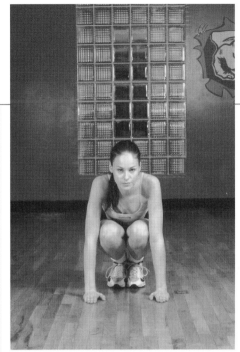

Squat with knees together and place hands on the floor in front of you. Lift your butt up while grasping your toes.

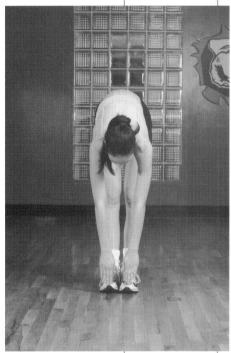

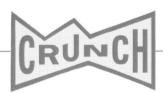

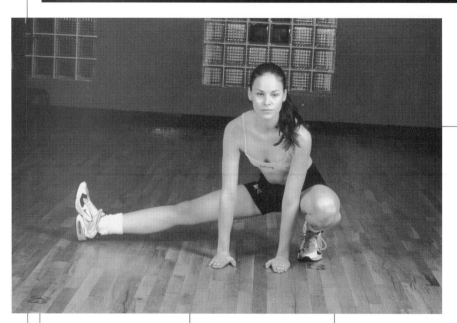

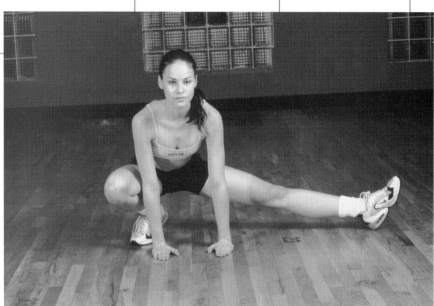

Standing with legs together, squat down. Fully extend right leg, putting hands flat on the floor. Your right heel should touch the ground. Don't hyperextend your knee. Hold for 10 seconds. Repeat on opposite side. Do two sets.

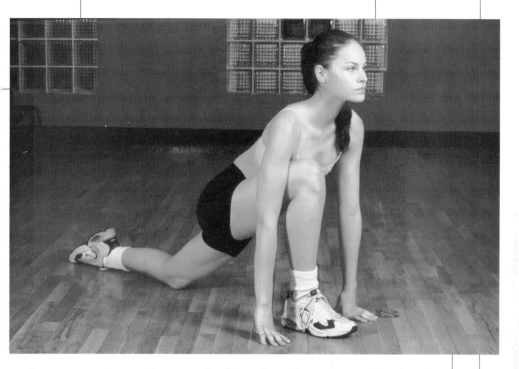

Lunge, putting one knee to the floor. Keep hips square. Put hands down and stretch forward, bringing chest down. Turn heel out. Repeat with opposite leg.

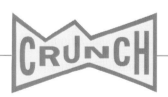

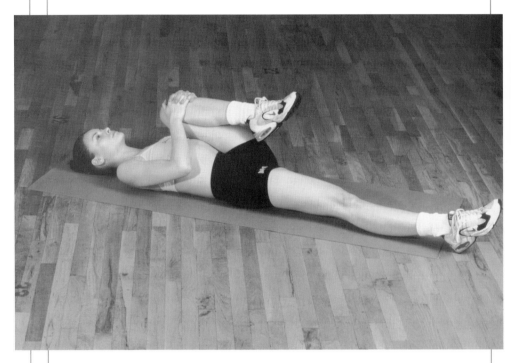

Lie on your back. Pull one leg up to your chest. Repeat with other leg.

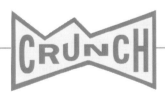

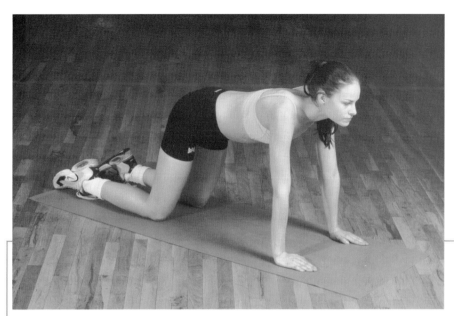

On all fours, bring your head down to the ground and stretch out your arms. This is a cat stretch.

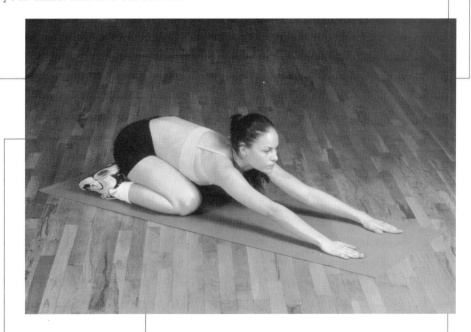

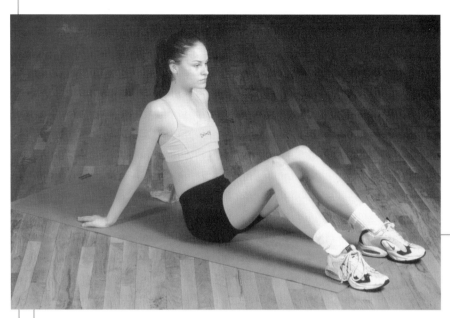

Flip over. With arms shoulder-length apart, hands on the floor with fingers pointing back, lift shoulders off ground and raise knees, keeping feet on floor. Keep your chest up. This is an M stretch.

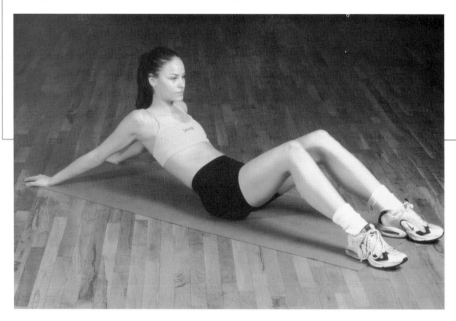

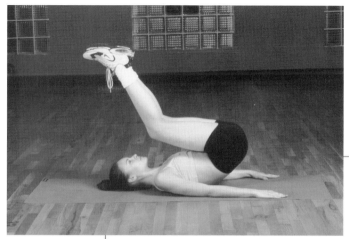

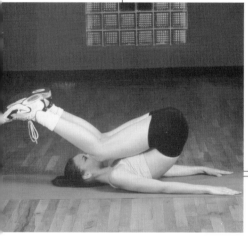

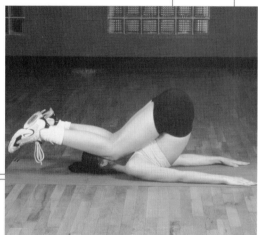

Lie down flat on your back. Kick legs over your head. Straddle your head, touch knees to the ground. Slowly roll legs back to the ground. Do twice.

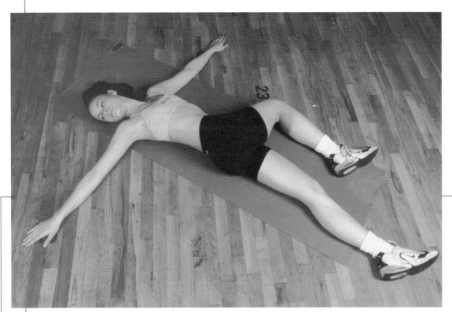

Lie flat on your back, with arms straight out to sides. Cross one leg over the other and turn head to look at opposite arm. Alternate sides. This is a good glute stretch. For a deeper stretch, change the height of the knee.

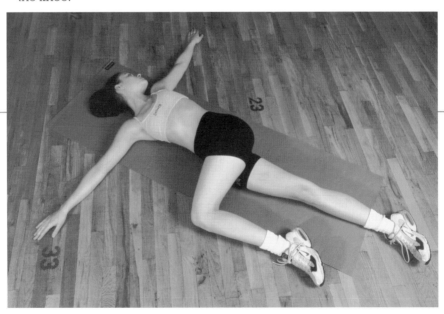

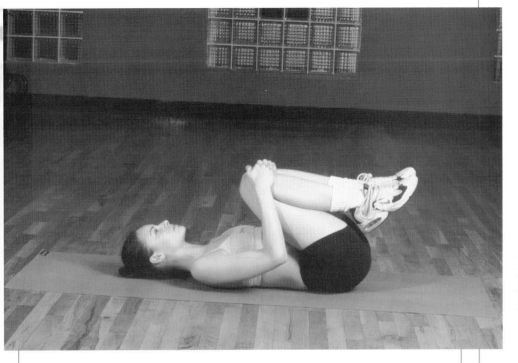

Lie on your back, grab your knees and pull them up to your chest.

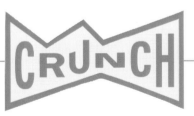

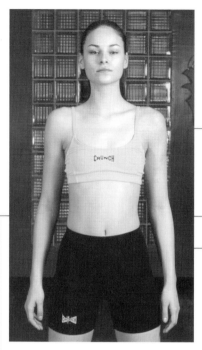 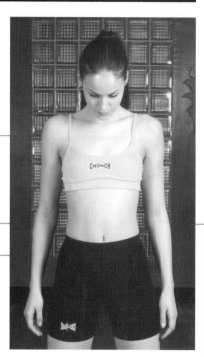

Do neck circles, but do not grind your neck *back*—it may damage your cartilage.

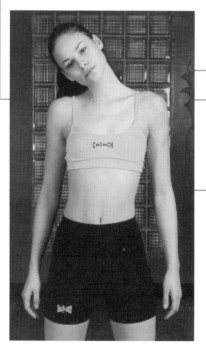 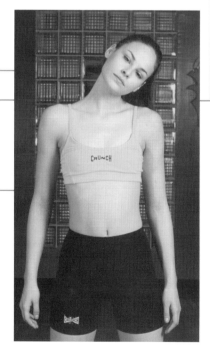

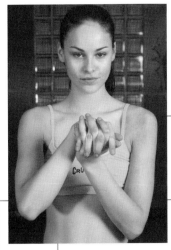

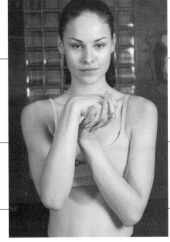

Clasp your hands together and rotate your wrist in circles.

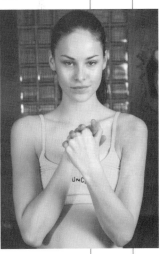

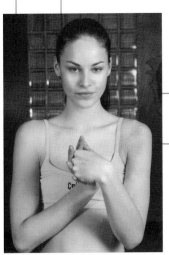

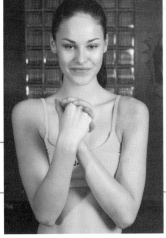

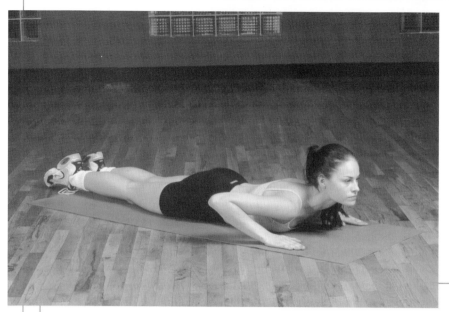

Lie on your stomach in the push-up position, and slowly push your chest up. Keep your hips on the ground and your neck back. This is a seal stretch.

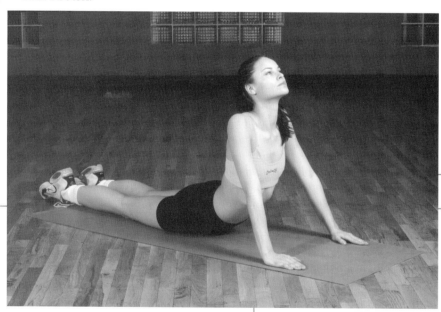

EARN YOUR WINGS ON THE GROUND

If there's one thing business travel is good for, it's accumulating frequent flyer miles that you can use for vacation travel. Of course, that means you must be able to consolidate all your business travel on one airline. The frequent flyer programs of the major U.S. airlines are fairly similar, but you may want to check out their Web sites to see which airline's schedules, amenities, destinations, and frequent flyer programs best suit you.

While it may seem as if those miles add up pretty quickly, frequent flyer programs typically require you to rack up over 25,000 miles before you can get a free ticket. As a result, most frequent flyer miles are redeemed for upgrades, rather than free tickets. However, there are plenty of ways to supplement your miles without leaving the ground. So if your heart is set on a free ticket to Australia (perhaps to run in the 2000 Olympic Marathon), or if you're short a few thousand miles to get that upgrade to first class, check with your airline to see what "affiliates" are part of its frequent flyer program. The most common affiliates, for example, are hotels and car rental agencies, but there are certainly others, such as:

- credit cards
- phone companies
- Dial-A-Mattress (American Airlines)
- 1-800-FLOWERS (United Airlines)
- car dealers (United)
- mortgage lenders (American)
- landscaping services (American)
- magazines (*Business Week*)
- charities (March of Dimes, Audobon Society, Jewish National Fund)

With such diverse ways to earn frequent flyer miles, you might be thinking, wouldn't it be great if I could earn frequent flyer miles at the gym? Well, CRUNCH understands how its road warrior members feel and has introduced Netpulse Stations in its gyms (see photo on next page). Each minute spent training on Netpulse equipment earns exercisers frequent flyer miles, free compact discs from Tower Records and Blockbuster Music, gift certificates to selected retailers, fantasy vacations, and other rewards. Netpulse Stations are ideal for busy professionals who barely have time to get to the gym—the technology allows exercisers to surf the Web, read an on-line newspaper or magazine, check sports scores, receive stock quotes and place trades, watch TV, listen to CDs, or even shop!

For more ways to earn free travel, here are some Web sites that offer specific tips for accumulating miles:

www.webflyer.com

(This site reviews and rates frequent flyer programs offered by major airlines, hotels, and credit cards.)

www.travelspots.com/trip_tips/ howto_earn_points.htm

http://members.aol.com/ffmiles

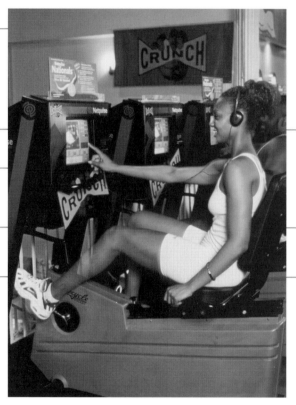

This road warrior has been pedalling for miles and miles . . . and frequent flyer miles.

PART 3
TRANQUILLITY IN TRANSIT

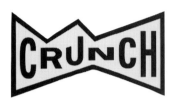

You don't have to be claustrophobic to panic at the mere idea of a long trip in a moving vehicle. Sitting in a cramped airline, train, or car seat for hours on end makes your muscles sore, your butt numb, and your mood nasty. Oh, to be able to stretch out your legs, put up your feet, throw your neighbor's carry-on bags across the aisle....

Just because you are allotted a tiny personal space for the trip's duration doesn't mean you can't stretch out. You just have to know which muscles need stretching in order to avoid soreness. Yoga happens to provide some very useful stretches. And with yoga, not only can you refresh your muscles, you can also refresh your mind.

You don't have to know a thing about yoga to perform the following moves and benefit from them. CRUNCH yoga instructor Sarah Ivanhoe has carefully chosen stretches that get your mind and body into the spirit of your trip. In fact, yoga is a very suitable activity for a trip. That's because yoga is all about taking a journey; it's not about the destination. Yogis believe life itself is a journey.

Practicing yoga represents a mythical quest. Hatha yoga was created as a means to approach spiritual enlightenment and to be completely in the present moment (it was *not* created just to get your body to do cool tricks). The word "hatha" has two components: "ha" means sun, and "tha" means moon. The sun represents fire or heat, and the moon represents coolness. By combining them in yoga, you achieve balance, which you need in order to move forward on your journey.

So as you board the plane, welcome yourself to your journey. Then, while you're in your seat and can't get up, consider doing some of the first few poses, which are good stretches for your shoulders.

STRETCHING AND RELAXATION POSES

1. Shoulder Rolls
2. Garudasana Arms (Eagle Pose)
3. Gomukasana Arms (Happy Cow Pose)
4. Parsvottanasana Arms (Reverse Namaste)
5. Uttita Hastasana
6. Shoulder Stretch
7. Ardha Chandrasana
8. Bidalasana
9. Neck Stretch
10. Knee to Chest
11. Thread the Needle
12. Lotus
13. Tolasana
14. Walking Meditation
15. Puppy Dog Pose
16. Dancer's Prep Pose
17. Hang Pose
18. Uttanasana

RESTORATIVE POSES

1. Restorative Pose #1
2. Restorative Pose #2
3. Meditation

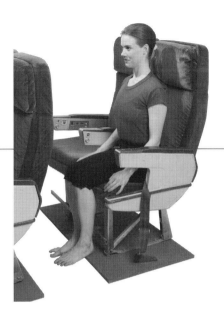

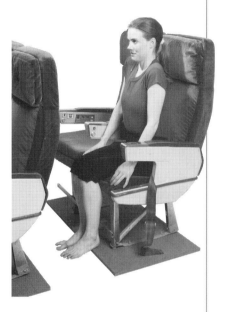

SHOULDER ROLLS

There are four directions the shoulders go in—forward, up, back, and down. Roll the shoulders clockwise, then counter clockwise. Try variations—one shoulder at a time, roll shoulders in opposite directions. Anyone can do this—no matter how old, or how out of shape you are. Shoulder rolls relieve tension, increase circulation, help posture, and reduce stress. You're actually giving yourself a little massage.

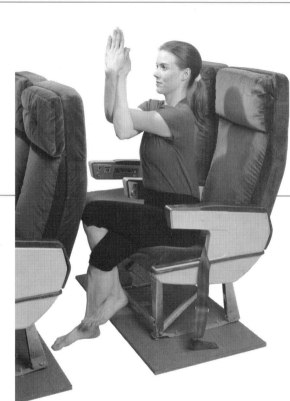

GARUDASANA ARMS
(Eagle Pose)

Start off your journey in an eagle pose, light and agile. The eagle is the king of the birds and represents graceful flight. This pose will prepare your mind and body to take flight.

Sitting in your chair, you're going to twine your arms and legs around each other. Put your right arm directly in front of you. Bend the right arm at the elbow, face your palm to the left, and point your thumb toward your head. Wrap your left arm all the way underneath the right arm, and swoop it around until your palms touch each other. Keep the shoulders down away from the ears. Lift the heart up to the ceiling and move the arms away from you — either up or down. Traditionally, you move the elbows down and the chest up, but play with it until your body finds the best stretch. Feel the stretch between the shoulder blades. Hold for at least one minute on each side. Breathe into the stretch while your shoulder blades (or wings) separate and stretch out. Open up your back, pulling everything away from the spine so your back is free and ready to move.

Concentration is essential for the pose—you're taking flight, and spreading your wings! Think of the shoulder blades as your wings, opening everything up and getting ready to take off.

GOMUKHASANA ARMS
(Happy Cow Pose)

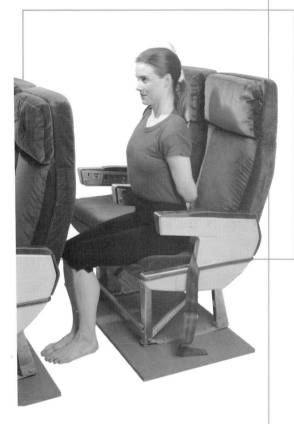

Lift your right arm up toward the ceiling, then bend your elbow and place your right hand on the base of the neck. The right elbow sticks up toward the ceiling. From the left side, hook the left palm facing away from your body and try to clasp your hands behind you. If the hands don't reach each other, grab onto a little towel or shirt (whatever's handy) so that each hand is holding something. (It's OK if the hands don't touch, but you do want to hold onto something.) Squeeze the right elbow straight back toward the chair and do the same with the left elbow. Make sure your lower belly is tucked in, your tailbone is down (taking it out of the lower back), and your sternum is lifted toward the stars. Perform this stretch on each side. Hold the pose for at least one minute.

It's beneficial to hold the stretch on one side for a minute or two, then fold it forward. Keep your arms exactly as they are—don't let the elbows flop to the side—and bring your chest to your thighs. Keep squeezing your elbows up.

This is a great shoulder stretch after you've been carrying luggage. The Gomukhasana does the opposite of what the first move did and stretches the shoulders in a different direction. It's called the "happy cow" pose because when the arms and legs are in the position, your body looks like the face of a smiling cow. Each bent elbow represents an ear, the belly button a nose, and the legs make a smile. It's one of the very few poses that represent a yogi's idea of a joke.

PARSVOTTANASANA ARMS (Reverse Namaste)

Namaste means "the divine within me salutes the divine within you." In spiritual terms, the reverse Namaste lifts up the body and spirit "by the bootstraps." And it's a great stretch for the shoulders.

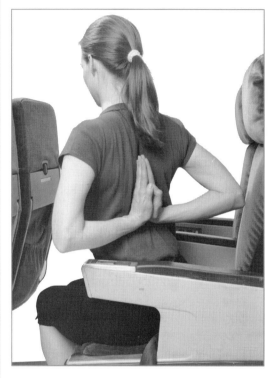

The Namaste pose is achieved by putting your palms in the prayer position at your heart. For reverse Namaste, bring the palms together on your back, with the fingertips pointing down. Bring fingertips into your back with palms together and flip them up. Try to walk the palms together and up your back. Your low belly should lift. Keeping your tailbone down, your heart lifts, and your shoulders move down away from your ears. Squeeze your shoulders and elbows together behind you. Men, beware: If you're not flexible enough, clasp your elbows behind you. You want to feel the chest lifting and shoulders squeezing back.

In this pose, your palms are directly behind your heart. This helps your heart lift up toward the sky, which sends your spirit up and out on your journey. If you can, hold this pose for five minutes. You may want to close your eyes and let your chin drop slightly (though keep your chest up) and use this pose for a meditation.

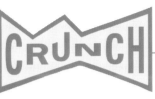

UTTITA HASTASANA

This pose is difficult! To get the arms really straight, you need to work your triceps like crazy. Very few people can actually do this stretch correctly. Bring your bellybutton into your body, your tailbone into the seat, and lift your chest. Do not sway your lower back. Interlace your fingers, press your palms toward the ceiling, and, staying soft in the jaw and neck, try to squeeze the arms straight. Squeeze elbows toward each other, pull outer edges of your arms forward, and then push them straight up through the palms.

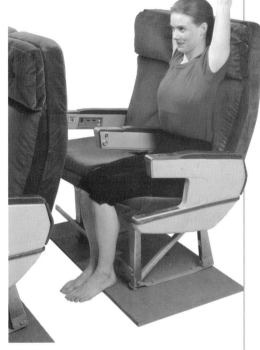

This stretch lengthens the sides of your body and is a real shoulder and arm strengthener, especially working the triceps. It will make you feel energized! The main line of energy in the body is the spine, and this stretch makes that line of energy longer. An energizing fire pose, this stretch gets people all fired up for the trip—do it as you're preparing to get off the plane.

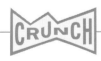

SHOULDER STRETCH

For this modern yoga move, interlace your fingers behind your back so your palms are touching. With your palms together, take both hands to the right side of your body. Try to pull your hands forward and squeeze your elbows and shoulders together behind you so you feel the heart lift and your lungs open. Make sure you stretch both sides. Hold for two minutes on each side. The longer you hold the pose, the better the stretch.

Like the reverse Namaste, this stretch opens the heart and lungs. It also helps to undo that hunched-over pro-

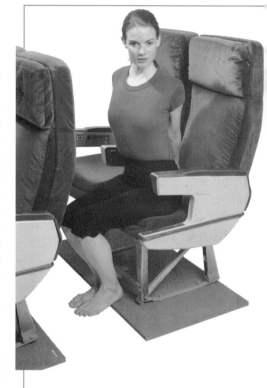

cess that happens to all of us. This pose isn't just stretching, it's restructuring the muscles in a way to combat kyphosis, that rounded hump in the back that comes with age. The emotional anatomy of people with a rounded upper back is that they are bearing the weight of the world on their shoulders. (Think of the Greek god Atlas.) Physiologically, the poor posture of rounded shoulders crushes the lungs and heart and creates an environment for disease.

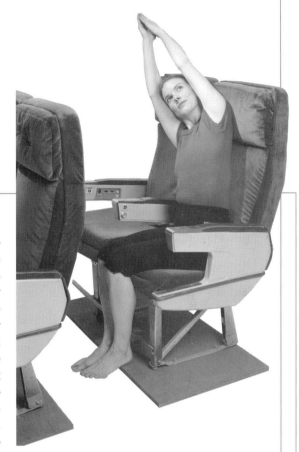

ARDHA CHANDRASANA
(Half-Moon Pose)

Lift your arms straight up over your head, with palms pressed together. Press your back and arms against the back of the chair. Keep your belly in, but bear in mind that there is a natural curve in the lower back, so don't worry if it doesn't touch the chair. Try to smoosh everything to the chairback. Reach up and over to the right. On the inhale, reach up to the sky and exhale over to the right a little more. Just go a couple of inches at a time so that you can identify the tight spots. When you find one, stay there and breathe until it softens. It is the breath that will encourage the tight spots to open. Don't collapse the chest...lift the heart. Repeat on the left.

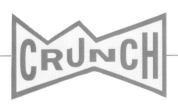

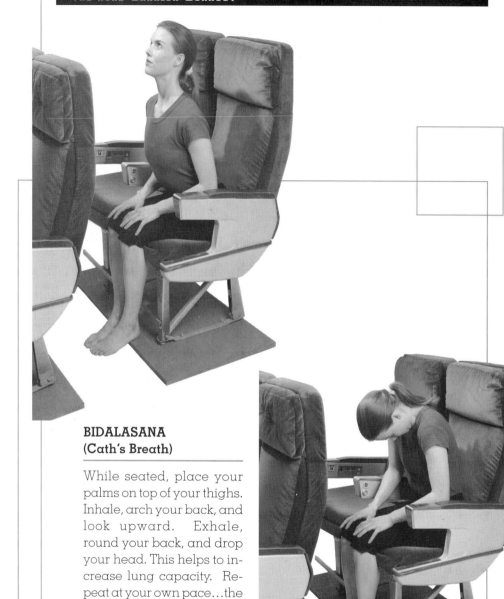

BIDALASANA
(Cath's Breath)

While seated, place your palms on top of your thighs. Inhale, arch your back, and look upward. Exhale, round your back, and drop your head. This helps to increase lung capacity. Repeat at your own pace...the slower the better. While fast movements are jarring to the spine, slow movements soothe and nourish the spine, gently encouraging it to become more fluid.

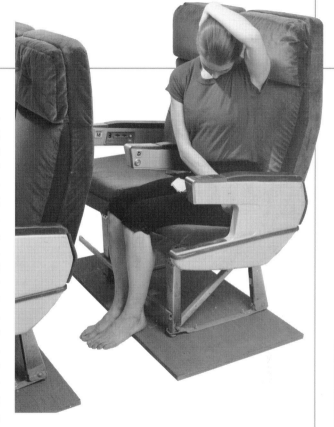

NECK STRETCH

A word about neck stretches: The muscles in your neck are very sensitive, so it's important to stretch them out gently and properly. With your right hand, grab onto the seat belt, where the belt meets the chair. Your body should be facing straight ahead. Position your chin over your left knee on a diagonal. Lift up your chest, and drop your head. Place your left hand on the right side of your neck and lean forward and toward the left. Feel an awesome stretch in the neck. Move an inch to the right or left to increase the stretch. When you have your right hand rooted there, your right shoulder is kept down and back. Holding onto the seat belt is the key! Repeat on the opposite side.

WALKING MEDITATION

Walk through the aisles of the plane slowly. Bring your mind into the present moment and pay close attention to how the sole of your foot feels on the floor. Ask yourself: Can I feel all five toes? Can I feel the foot move from the heel to the toe? Step forward on the exhale and use each step as a breath. Use each step as a step toward inner peace. When you notice your mind wandering, bring your attention back to your feet and your breathing.

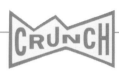

PUPPY DOG POSE

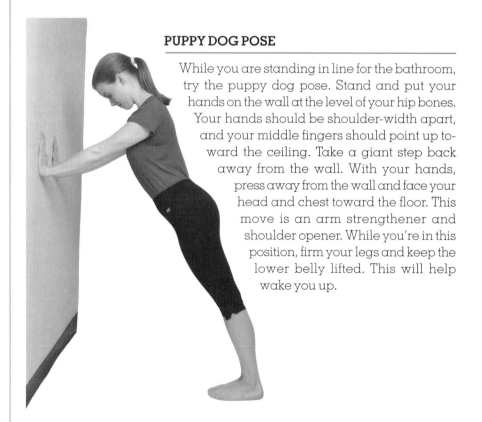

While you are standing in line for the bathroom, try the puppy dog pose. Stand and put your hands on the wall at the level of your hip bones. Your hands should be shoulder-width apart, and your middle fingers should point up toward the ceiling. Take a giant step back away from the wall. With your hands, press away from the wall and face your head and chest toward the floor. This move is an arm strengthener and shoulder opener. While you're in this position, firm your legs and keep the lower belly lifted. This will help wake you up.

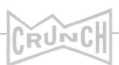

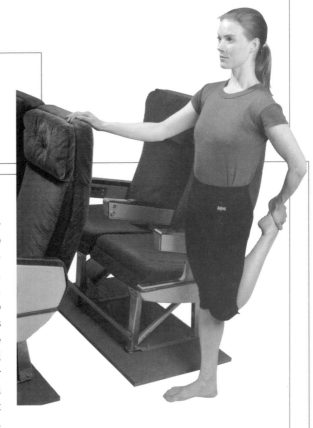

DANCER'S PREP POSE

With one hand, hold onto something to steady yourself. With the other hand, reach back behind you, grab onto your foot, and go for the quad stretch. (This is one stretch that everyone hates to do, so now's a good time to get it in!) Keep your knees in line with each other. Don't let the bent knee flop out to the side. Keep your belly in and tailbone down so that when you're pulling your foot back, you're not doing a lower back stretch. Keeping your belly in and squeezing your butt down toward the floor aims the stretch right where it counts. This is an excellent stretch because plane travel can affect circulation in the legs—this stretch will wake them up. Repeat with the other leg.

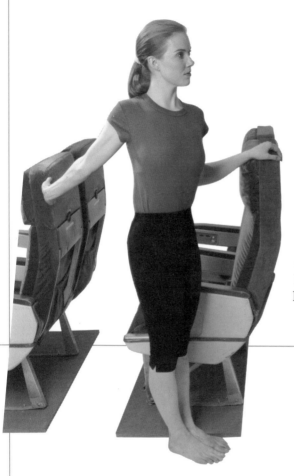

HANG POSE

This is a great stretch for the pectoral muscles. With one hand, grab onto your seat back—the doorway between first class and coach—and rotate your body away from your hand. Repeat on the opposite side.

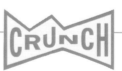

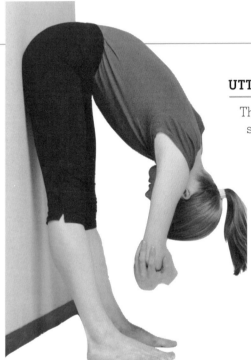

UTTANASANA

This stretch works the hamstrings and helps to relieve tension from the head, neck, back, and shoulders. Grasping your elbows, stand with your back against the wall and fall forward. Place your sit bones against the wall and keep your feet four to six inches apart, and four to six inches away from the wall. When your sit bones are against the wall, the effect is very grounding.

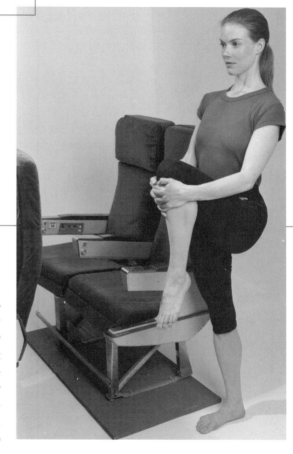

KNEE TO CHEST

While standing, hug one knee into your chest. This stretches out the lower back and the hips. It's very good for your digestion, massaging the internal organs. It's especially good to do during a flight, which causes constipation in many people. It helps to squeeze everything down and out. Do this stretch on each side, as many times as you want.

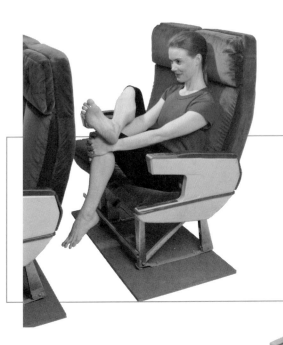

THREAD THE NEEDLE

While sitting in your seat, put your feet flat on the floor so that your lower legs are perpendicular to your upper legs. Take the outside of your right ankle and place it onto your left knee. Hug your left knee into your chest. Move your left knee toward your body, and squeeze your right knee away from the body. Keep flexing your right foot—point your right toes toward your right knee in order to protect the knee joint. If you feel any discomfort in the knee at all...stop!! Move the foot one inch up or down and try it again. If you cannot do the stretch without experiencing knee pain, then *try another stretch*.

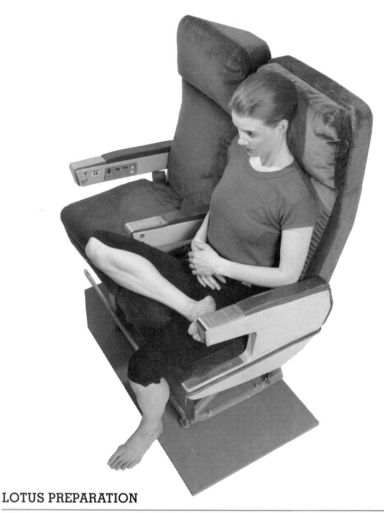

LOTUS PREPARATION

Bring your right foot all the way up to where the leg meets the body—at the groin. Squeeze the right knee down toward the floor. That's a half lotus, which you can do on each side. The size of your airline seat will probably prohibit you from achieving a full lotus position, but that's OK. Remember, yoga is about taking the journey, not the destination.

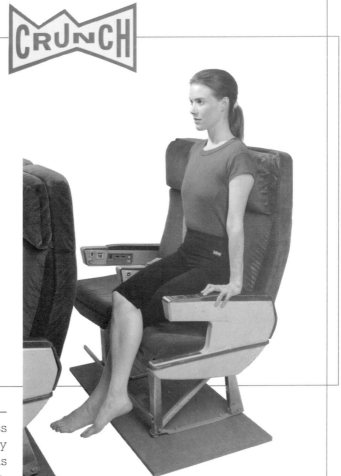

TOLASANA

While seated, cross your legs comfortably and put your hands on the armrests. Straighten your arms and push your body up. The goal in this move, ultimately, is to come off the seat, but it's a very hard move to do. Keep trying! It doesn't matter if you actually make it—it's the effort along the way that will make you stronger.

THE FOLLOWING MOON POSES CULTIVATE THE RESTORATIVE AND COOLING ASPECTS OF YOGA.

RESTORATIVE POSES

In restorative poses the weight of the body is supported so you can surrender your weight completely. The benefits go through the entire body, but you're not pulling, pushing, or tugging for the effects. You're actually able to relax.

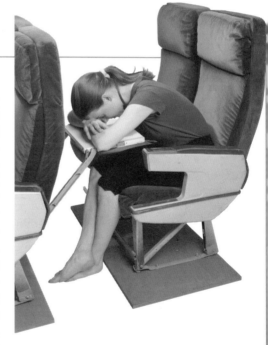

RESTORATIVE POSE #1

Lower the tray table and fold your arms on top of it. Put your forehead on your over-lapped wrists and get comfortable. Relax. Bend forward and allow your upper body weight to be supported. Any forward bend is good for the back, the face, and the jaw. Even though it looks as though you're not doing any-thing, learning to relax is a skill that we develop—like any other skill—by practice, practice, practice! Cross your arms over the tray, put your head down on your arms, and let go . . .

Try practicing the art of relaxing. Concentrate on relaxation—calming the mind and body—whenever possible so you can become really good at it!

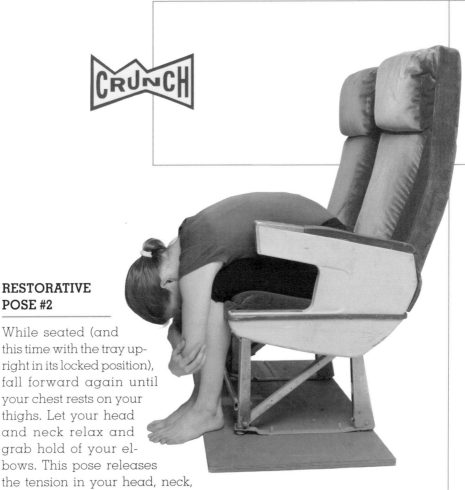

RESTORATIVE POSE #2

While seated (and this time with the tray upright in its locked position), fall forward again until your chest rests on your thighs. Let your head and neck relax and grab hold of your elbows. This pose releases the tension in your head, neck, jaw, and face. When you let go of the tension, you have all that energy left over to use for whatever you need it for. If you spend all your energy gripping your head, neck, and jaw, you get off the plane having spent that energy. One of the things yoga can teach you is to learn how to focus your energy so that you can put it to use where you want to. If you feel silly folded forward, reach around with your hand and pretend to look for something!

MEDITATION

Meditation involves bringing your mind into the present moment. For the first meditation, we're going to focus on breathing using a zipassana technique. With the eyes closed, on the inhale mentally say, "in" and on the exhale mentally say "out." It sounds simple, but it's actually one of the hardest things you'll ever try to do. Do about four breaths, and when you notice your mind starting to drift off, come back and silently repeat "in" and "out." Yoga is defined as the restraining of the modifications of the mind. That's what you're doing when you're meditating. When your mind is racing with thoughts about the connections you have to catch and all the work you have to do and whether you remembered to pack such and such, it's going into a thousand other places, which scatters your energy. A focused mind will focus that energy in order to spend it how and where you want. Meditating brings you back to the present moment. It is a present moment that helps settle us and ultimately set us free.

As you disembark the plane, you should feel relaxed yet energized—and mentally focused for your work ahead.

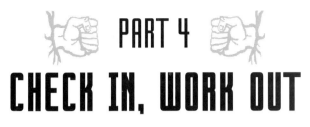

PART 4
CHECK IN, WORK OUT

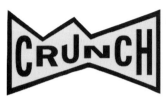

Face it, business travelers don't usually get to stay at the Ritz. But whether you're staying at a Marriott or a Motel 6, the condition of—or lack of—the hotel's fitness facilities shouldn't concern you. That's because you don't need a fully equipped gym at your hotel to get a thorough workout. For this hotel room workout, all you need are a jumprope, an exercise band, and a bath towel.

As we reviewed in the Pre-Travel Workout, for a workout to be complete, it must contain the following components—aerobic, strength, and flexibility.

Cardiovascular exercise improves the heart and lungs, bringing oxygenated blood to all the working muscles. It also helps burn fat. Also known as aerobic exercise, it helps to burn fat. During aerobic exercise your body continuously delivers oxygen to your muscles. It is during aerobic exercise that your body uses fat as its primary fuel source.

The jumprope is the cheapest piece of cardio equipment and is portable enough to throw right into the suitcase. It helps to strengthen the quads, calves, hamstrings, and forearms. A great form of cardio, jump roping allows you to burn up to 300 calories in a 30-minute workout.

This hotel room workout is based on circuit training. You will move quickly from exercise to exercise with little or no rest at all. Although it may feel as though you are working aerobically, the workout is more precisely defined as strength training. However, after you finish the circuit, you can go back to the jumprope for another 20 minutes of cardio exercise.

Strength training builds strong muscles, which help protect the bones and support the joints. For this part of the workout, you'll be using your own body weight, an exercise band, and your luggage to create resistance.

Flexibility training improves your range of motion through the joints and reduces the risk of injury. Stretching is the key to maintaining flexibility.

The exercise band is versatile and great for traveling. It's a nice change from cold, steel dumbbells and big pieces of machinery. Exercise bands come in varying tensions. The heavier the band, the more muscle strength is needed.

THE HOTEL ROOM WORKOUT

Think your room is just for sleeping? Think again. It's a full-service gym as well. In the following workout, you'll be setting up a "circuit" in the room.

HOTEL ROOM WORKOUT

Exercise	Reps (or time duration)	
Jumprope Warm-up	6	minutes
One-Leg Squats	15–20	
Lunges	15–20	each leg
Push-ups	10–15	
Jump Rope	3	minutes
Tricep Dips	10–15	
Hip Extensions	20–25	
Ski Hops	60	seconds
90 Second Wall-sits	90	seconds
Tricep Pressdowns	15	
Bicep Curls	15	
One-Arm Rows	15	
Upright Rows	12–15	
Anterior Raises	12–15	
Jump Rope	90	seconds
Crescent Kicks	20–25	each leg
Table Chin-ups	10–12	
Crunches	20–25	
Hyper-Extensions	6–10	per side
Cool-down		

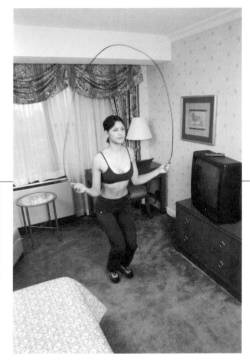

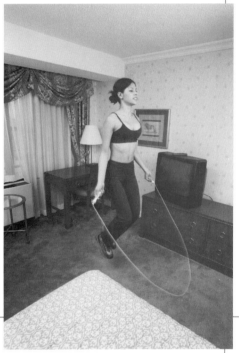

Begin by jumping rope for 6 minutes to allow your body to warm up. Warming up is very important before any type of workout. It increases the temperature in your muscles and makes the joints more pliable and less likely to tear. It begins to increase the blood flow to working muscles, providing an increasing supply of oxygen.

Hotel room courtesy of Holiday Inn— Midtown, New York.

Next, move over to the dresser and remove the bottom drawer for squats, lunges, and push-ups.

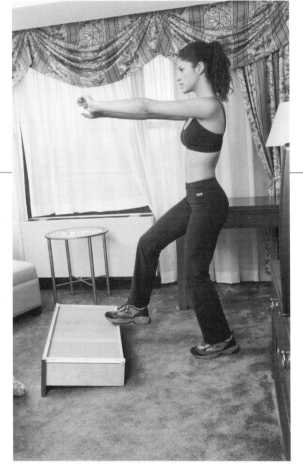

ONE-LEG SQUATS

Stand with legs hip-distance apart, keeping your knees "soft" and maintaining good posture. Step back with your right foot and keep it planted firmly on the floor. Next, place your left heel on the dresser and make sure your knees are slightly bent. Bring your arms forward for balance. Keep your chest up and slowly lower your hips as if you were sitting in a chair. Rise without locking your knees and repeat 15 to 20 times. From this stance, pivot and turn your body around, preparing for lunges.

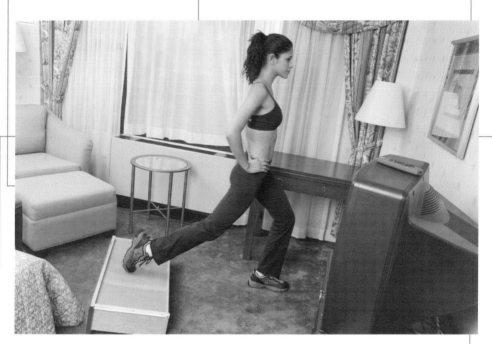

LUNGES

First, check your body alignment. The ball of the left foot should be on the dresser drawer. The left hip should be aligned with the left knee. The right knee should be aligned with the right foot. Keep your chest up and lower your hips toward the floor to a comfortable position. Squeeze your glutes and rise without locking your knees. To maintain proper alignment the front knee should stay in line with the foot throughout the exercise. Repeat 15 to 20 times. Switch legs and repeat another 15 to 20 times.

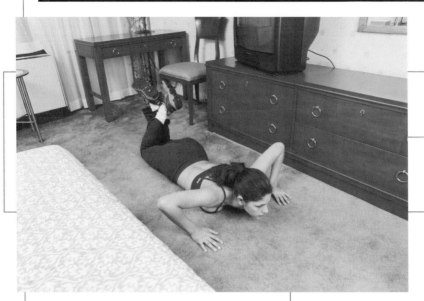

PUSH-UPS

The push-up mainly targets the chest, but also tones the triceps and deltoids. Although most people refer to the push-up as an upper-body exercise, the lower body and abdominal muscles are worked by helping to stabilize the body during the exercise. Start by lying flat on the floor face down. Place your hands on the floor by the side of your chest. Cross your ankles and bend the knees. Line up the neck and spine all the way down to the knees. Take a deep breath and as you exhale, push your body up without locking the 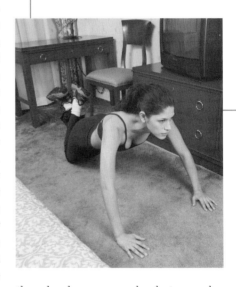 elbows. Inhale, and as you tighten the abs, lower your body toward the floor, bending from the elbows and bringing your chest toward the floor. Repeat 10 to 15 times. To make this more challenging, extend your legs and balance on your toes.

Jump rope again for 3 minutes. Upon completion, move over to the desk chair for some tricep dips and hip extensions.

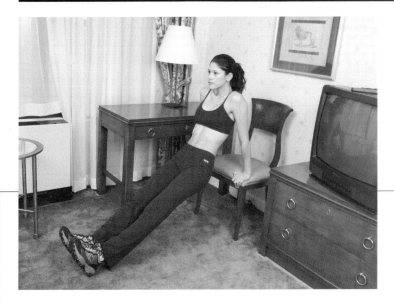

TRICEP DIPS

Dips target the back of the arms and rear deltoid. Place the chair against the wall to steady it, and sit on the chair with your legs extended. Grasp the end of the chair with fingertips facing forward and slide your butt off the chair. Lower yourself toward the floor by bending at your elbows. Straighten your arms again to complete the movement, but don't let your elbows lock. Repeat 10 to 15 times.

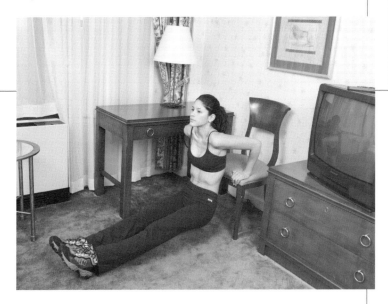

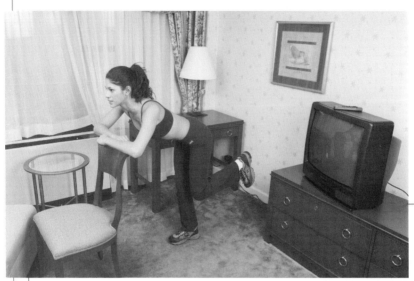

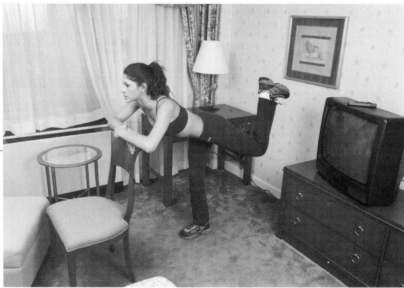

HIP EXTENSIONS

These work the glutes and hamstrings. Stand behind the chair and bend forward at the hips and fold your arms over the chair. Align your head, neck, and spine. Pull your abs in tight to support your lower back. Next, raise the right leg so that the knee is at a 90 degree angle, and keep your left leg slightly bent. Flex your foot and press your heel up toward the ceiling until the right thigh is parallel to the floor. Squeeze your glutes at the top of the movement and lower your leg. Repeat 20 to 25 times and switch legs.

GET THE DRESSER DRAWER OUT FOR SOME SKI HOPS

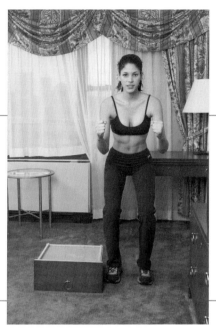

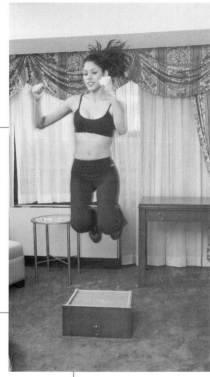

SKI HOPS

This is a great exercise for the lower body and a perfect shot of cardio and strength. We're going to start on one side of the dresser with the legs bent and a neutral spine (good posture). From here, leap over the drawer to the other side, landing on both feet with the knees slightly bent. Feel free to use your arms to help lift you off the floor. If your dresser drawer is too wide, use your imagination—you can use your suitcase or even a towel. Continue for 60 seconds (approximately 25 jumps side to side).

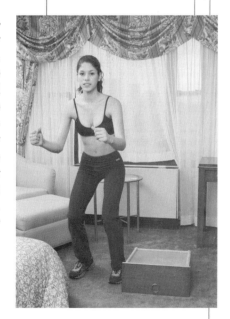

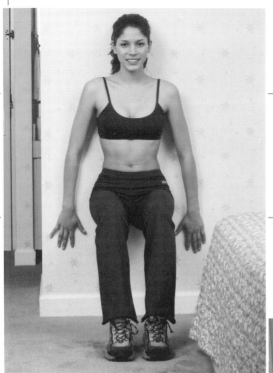

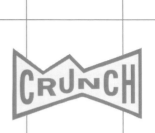

90-SECOND WALL SITS

Another great strength-
ener for the lower body.
Keeping your back up
against the wall, walk your
feet out and slide down.
"Sit" with your hips and
your knees at 90 degree
angles. Keep your shoul-
ders, head, and butt
against the wall. Pull the
abs in and hold this position for 90 seconds. Do not
be discouraged if you have
to stop before 90 seconds.
Just try again.

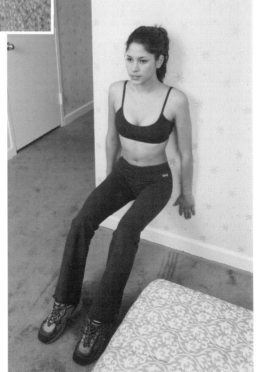

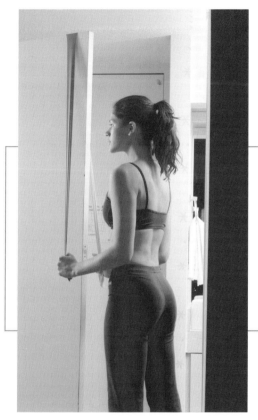

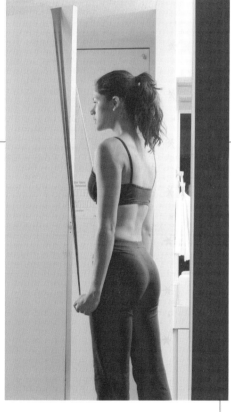

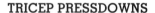

TRICEP PRESSDOWNS

Move to the closet and drape the exercise band evenly over the door. Stand close to the door and wrap the ends of the band around each hand. Start with your arms bent, by your sides, with your palms facing the floor. The only things that should move are your forearms as you pull the band down toward the floor, fully extending your arms without locking your elbows. Repeat 15 times.

Remove the exercise band from the door, place it underneath your feet, wrap the end of the band in each hand and get ready for some bicep curls.

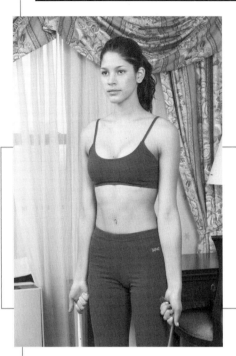
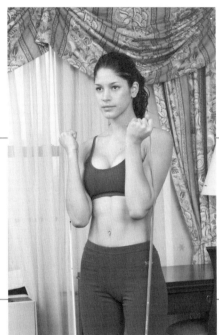

BICEP CURLS

Stand on the middle of the exercise band with your feet hip-distance apart. Keep your abs pulled in and your spine straight. With your arms down at your sides, and palms facing forward, hold an end of the band in each hand. Bend your elbows and curl both arms upward until your hands are in front of your shoulders. Lower your arms in a slow, controlled movement. If there is not enough resistance, wrap the band around each hand. Repeat 15 times.

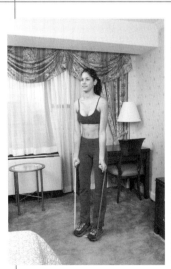
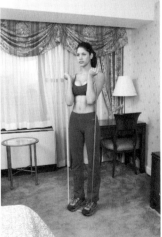

Jump rope for 90 seconds.

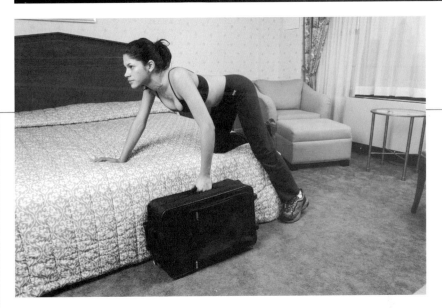

ONE-ARM ROWS WITH THE SUITCASE

One-arm rows target the lattisimus dorsi (large muscle of the back) and the biceps. Rest your left knee and left hand on the foot of the bed and flex forward from the hips so your back is flat. Hold the suitcase in the right hand and let the arm hang straight down from the shoulder. Draw elbow up toward the ceiling by squeezing the shoulder blade toward the spine. Lower slowly and repeat 15 times. Switch sides.

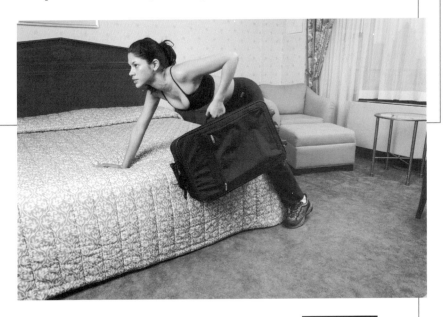

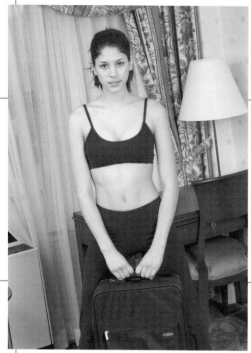

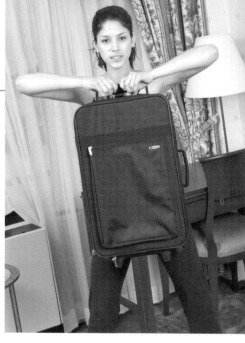

UPRIGHT ROWS WITH SUITCASE

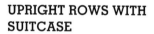

Upright rows target the upper part of the back (trapezius) and the rear deltoid, which aids good posture. To start, stand straight with feet a little wider than hip-distance apart. Place your hands together on the suit-case handle (think thumbs together). Raise the suitcase to mid-chest, beneath your chin with your elbows out to the side, squeezing the shoulder blades together. Imagine you are drawing a line from your belly button to your chin. Draw your hands closer to your body at the top. Lower in a slow and controlled motion. Repeat 12 to 15 times. To increase resistance, just weigh down the suitcase!

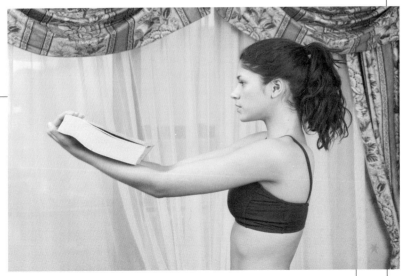

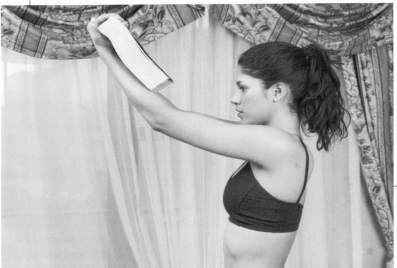

ANTERIOR RAISE WITH A HOTEL DIRECTORY

This move targets the anterior deltoid and biceps. Stand straight with good posture, knees slightly bent. Turn palms up. Place the phone book in the palms of your hands. Raise the arms to shoulder level with elbows slightly bent. Now raise your arms approximately 2 to 3 inches from shoulder level and return to shoulder level. Repeat 12 to 15 times.

Jump rope for 90 seconds.

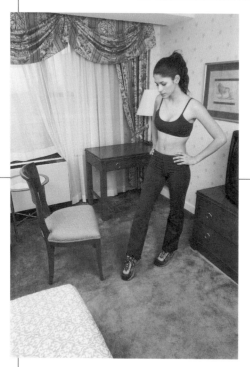

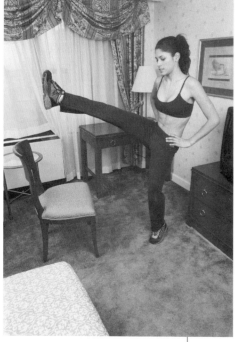

CRESCENT KICKS

This exercise works the inner and outer thighs as well as the glutes and abs. Plus, it's good for overall balance because you will be standing on one leg. Stand in front of the chair, with your legs wider than hip-distance apart. Start with the right leg. Sweep it over the chair in a half-circle motion, creating the shape of a crescent moon. Keep your arms by your sides and pull your abs in for balance. Start with the crescent kick over the seat of the chair. If you find this too easy, turn the chair around. Repeat 20 to 25 times and switch legs

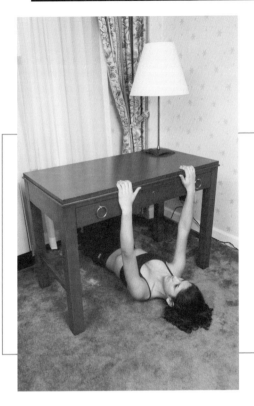

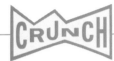

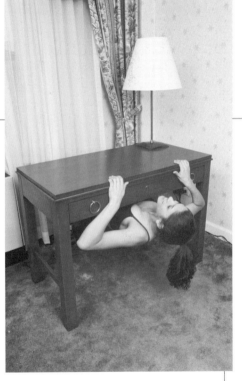

TABLE CHIN-UPS

These chin-ups target the lattisimus dorsi (back), the biceps, and the forearms. Move over to the desk and lie on your back with your legs underneath the table top. Bend your knees bent and place your feet flat on the floor. Grasp the edge of the desk with your arms almost fully extended. At this point, check your grip—if the table surface is slick with polish, your grip may slip easily. Also, make sure the table is sturdy enough that you won't pull it over!

If the table is safe, bend your elbows to pull your chin toward the desk top. Keep your back straight and your chin up. Lower in a slow, controlled motion. Repeat 10 to 12 times.

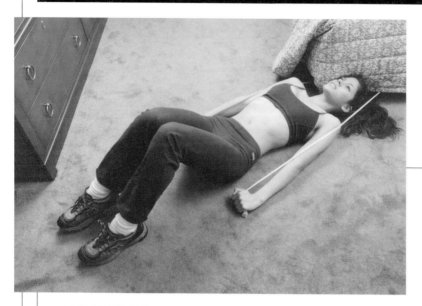

ABDOMINALS

Wrap the exercise band evenly around the leg of the bed. Lie on your
back with your feet pointing away from the bed. Wrap each end of
the band around each hand and place your hands by your sides,
palms facing down. Take a deep breath, and, as you exhale, crunch
your abdominals to lift your head and shoulders inches off the ground.
For variation, lift your feet off the ground. To target the obliques, add
trunk twists. As you crunch, bring one hand toward the opposite knee.

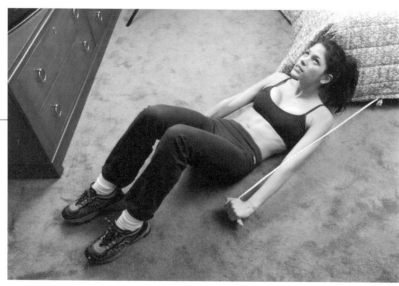

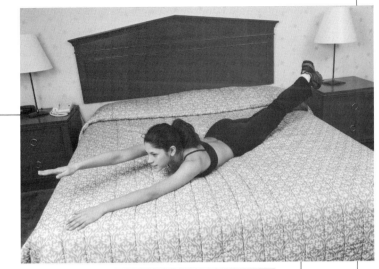

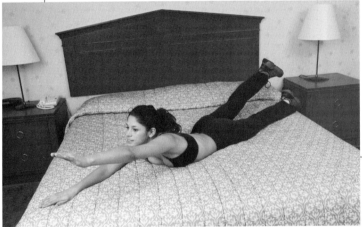

HYPER-EXTENSION

This move targets the erector spinae (muscles of the lower back). It's important to include exercises for the lower back, which is often neglected in most workout routines. We spend a lot of time focusing on abs to develop strength and, of course, flatten the stomach, but we must remember to work opposing muscle groups equally to avoid imbalances, that could lead to injury.

Lie face down on the bed and stretch your arms straight above your head, and extend your legs 2 to 3 inches apart. Keep your shoulder blades down and together. Lift your right leg and the left arm in a slow, controlled movement. Hold for 5 seconds and lower. Imagine lifting up and lengthening out the torso. Repeat 6 to 10 times and then switch the arm and leg.

COOL DOWN

Have you worked up a sweat? Good job! Grab your towel and wipe yourself down. Next, roll the towel up the long way. We're going to use it for stretching.

Hold each stretch for approximately 30 to 60 seconds.

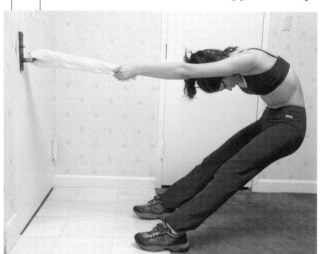

For the back and torso: Wrap the towel around the bedpost (or something sturdy). Hold one end of the towel in each hand. Facing the bed with your arms fully extended, lean back, flexing forward from your hips.

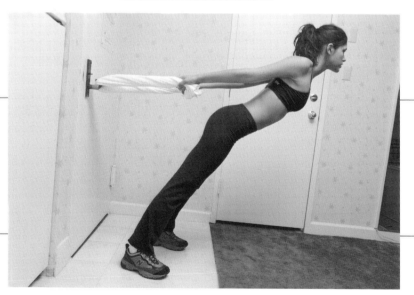

For the chest and shoulders: This is the opposite of the first stretch. Hold one end of the towel in each hand. Facing away from the bed, lean forward, flexing from the hips.

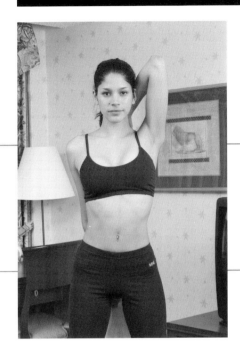

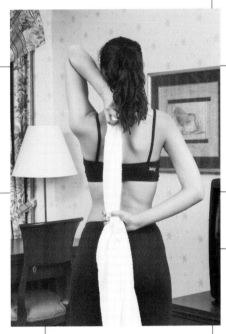

For the triceps: Stand with good posture, feet hip-width apart. Hold one end of the towel in each hand. Place your right hand near the small of your back and extend your left arm over your head. Gently pull with your right hand on the towel so that your left elbow bends, allowing your left hand to reach toward your left shoulder. Keep your left elbow pointing toward the ceiling. Switch arms.

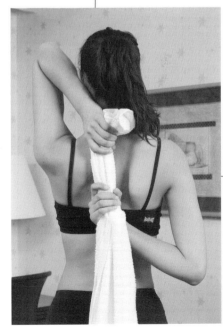

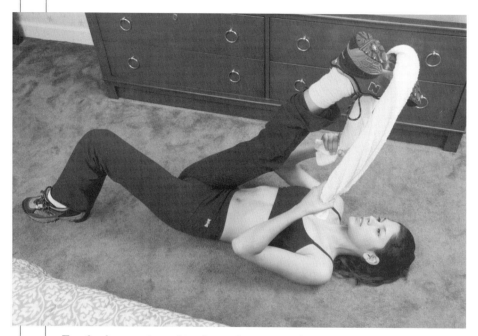

For the hamstrings: Lie down face up with your left knee bent and left foot on the floor. Wrap the towel around your right foot while holding one end of the towel in each hand. Fully extend your right leg up so that the bottom of the foot is facing the ceiling. Now pull the towel gently toward your torso until you feel a slight tension in the back of the leg. Repeat on the left side.

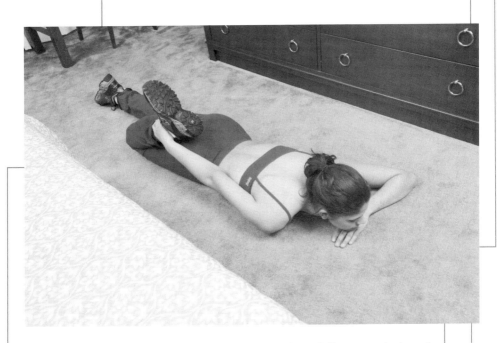

For the quadriceps: Lie face down with your legs fully extended and hands under your chin. Bend your right knee, bringing your right foot toward your butt. Reach for your foot with your right hand and gently pull your foot closer to the glutes. Flex your foot. Repeat on the left side.

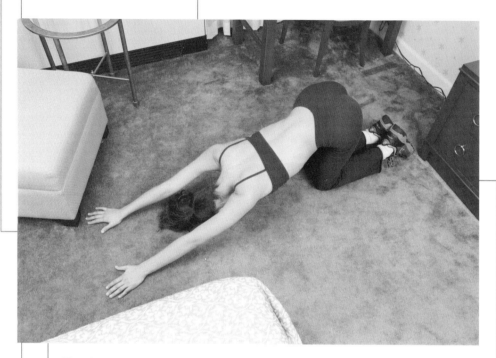

For the hips, abs, and upper body: Position yourself on your hands and knees. Align your shoulders with your elbows and your hips with your knees. Slide your hands forward over your head so your torso forms one long line from your hips to your fingertips. Lower your torso until your forehead is touching the floor, keeping your hips up and aligned with your knees.

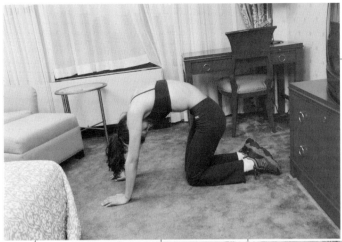

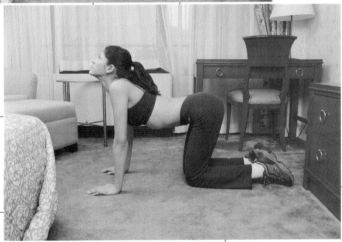

For your lower back and abdominals: Position yourself on your hands and knees. Keep your back flat and in alignment with your neck and head. Pull your abdominals in and round your back, dropping your chin into your chest. Hold for a count of 5 and then release, putting a slight arch in your spine and lifting your chin up toward the ceiling. (This is a cat stretch.)

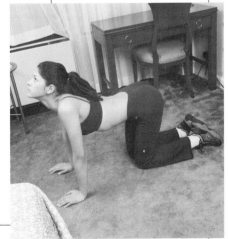

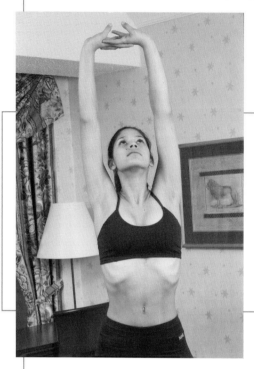

Stand, take a deep breath in, and bring your arms overhead. Clasp your hands together, palms up, and reach a little higher toward the ceiling. Exhale and lower your arms.

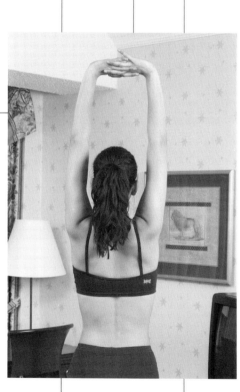

That's it—now you can hit the shower!

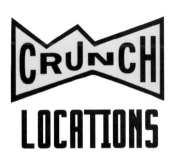

LOCATIONS

Where to work out, pretend to work out, or just stand around calling our personal trainers "Hans" and "Franz" under your breath.

NEW YORK CITY

404 Lafayette Street
(Astor Place and 4th Avenue)
212.614.0120

152 Christopher Street
(at Greenwich Street)
212.366.3725

54 East 13th Street
(University and Broadway)
212.475.2018

1109 Second Avenue
(at 59th Street)
212.758.3434

162 West 83rd Street
(Columbus and Amsterdam)
212.875.1902

144 W. 38th St.
(7th Ave. & Broadway)
212.869.7788

623 Broadway (at Houston)
212.420.0507

LOS ANGELES

8000 Sunset Blvd.
(West Hollywood)
323.654.4550

SAN FRANCISCO

1000 Van Ness Avenue
(Geary and O'Farrell)
415.931.1100

MISSION VIEJO

The Kaleidoscope Center
27741 Crown Valley Parkway
949.582.8181

MIAMI

1259 Washington Avenue
(South Beach)
305.674.8222

ATLANTA AREA
[ALL LOCATIONS: 800.660.5433]

Crunch Club Cobb
North by NW Office Park
1775 Water Place
Atlanta, GA 30339

Crunch Gwinnett
Gwinnett Prado
2300 Pleasant Hill Road
Duluth, GA 30136

Crunch Town Center
Main Street Shopping Center
2600 Prado Lane
Marietta, GA 30066

Crunch Roswell
Roswell Exchange
11060 Alpharetta Highway
Roswell, GA 30076

Crunch Buckhead
3365 Piedmont Road, Suite 1010
Atlanta, GA

Crunch Stone Mountain
Stone Mountain Square
5370 Highway 78 South
Stone Mountain, GA 30087

TOKYO

Crunch Omotesando
4-3-24 Jingumae Sibuya

Coming soon to Las Vegas and Chicago!

Visit us on the Web at
www.crunch.com

Have questions about this workout?

Ask the authors at:

WWW.GETFITNOW.COM

*The **hottest** fitness spot on the internet!*

FEATURING . . .

"Ask the Expert" Q&A Boards

Stimulating Discussion groups

Cool Links

Great Photos

Full-Motion Videos

Downloads

The Five Star Fitness Team

Hot Product Reviews

And More!

Log on today to receive a FREE catalog
or call us at
1-800-906-1234

Fit Test / Personal Training Session

15% OFF! 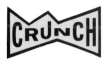 15% OFF!

IT'S EASY . . . Come into any CRUNCH location and receive 15% off your first purchase of personal training. Then just sign, date, and present this coupon at the fitness desk to set up your session.

MEMBER NAME	SIGNATURE

TRAINER NAME	TRAINER SIGNATURE

DATE OF SESSION

Cannot be combined with any other offer. Valid for one use only

- - - - - - - - - - - - CUT AT DOTTED LINE - - - - - - - - - - -

GUEST PASS

$22 value!

Must show picture ID to use facility.
The same guest may use only two guest passes per year

MEMBERSHIP REP	EXPIRATION DATE

OUR MISSION AND PHILOSOPHY

We at CRUNCH warmly welcome people from all walks of life,
regardless of shape, size, sex, or ability.
People don't have to be flawless to feel at home at CRUNCH. We don't care
if our members are 18 or 80, fat or thin, short or tall, muscular or mushy, blond or bald,
or anywhere in between. CRUNCH is not competitive, it is non-judgmental,
it is not elitist, it does not represent a kind of person.
CRUNCH is a gym; a movement which is growing as we continue to perfect our ability
to create an environment where our members don't feel self-conscious,
and don't worry about what others think.
At the heart of CRUNCH's core stands a tremendously experienced and energetic staff
dedicated to creating an environment where everyone feels accepted—
a truly unique place!

WWW.CRUNCH.COM

*The **hottest** fitness spot on the internet!*

OUR MISSION AND PHILOSOPHY

We at CRUNCH warmly welcome people from all walks of life,
regardless of shape, size, sex, or ability.
People don't have to be flawless to feel at home at CRUNCH. We don't care
if our members are 18 or 80, fat or thin, short or tall, muscular or mushy, blond or bald,
or anywhere in between. CRUNCH is not competitive, it is non-judgmental,
it is not elitist, it does not represent a kind of person.
CRUNCH is a gym; a movement which is growing as we continue to perfect our ability
to create an environment where our members don't feel self-conscious,
and don't worry about what others think.
At the heart of CRUNCH's core stands a tremendously experienced and energetic staff
dedicated to creating an environment where everyone feels accepted—
a truly unique place!

WWW.CRUNCH.COM

*The **hottest** fitness spot on the internet!*

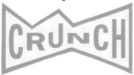

- - - - - - - - - - - CUT AT DOTTED LINE - - - - - - - - - - -

NEW YORK CITY

404 Lafayette Street
(Astor Place and 4th Street)
212.614.0120

54 East 13th Street
(University and Broadway)
212.475.2018

162 West 83rd Street
(Columbus and Amsterdam)
212.875.1902

623 Broadway (at Houston)
212.420.0507

152 Christopher Street
(at Greenwich Street)
212.366.3725

1109 Second Avenue
(at 59th Street)
212.758.3434

144 W. 38th St.
(7th Ave. & Broadway)
212.869.7788

LOS ANGELES

8000 Sunset Blvd.
(West Hollywood)
323.654.4550

SAN FRANCISCO

1000 Van Ness Avenue
(Geary and O'Farrell)
415.931.1100

MISSION VIEJO

The Kaleidoscope Center
27741 Crown Valley
  Parkway
949.582.8181

MIAMI

1259 Washington Avenue
(South Beach)
305.674.8222

ATLANTA AREA
(All locations: 800.660.5433)

Crunch Club Cobb
North by NW Office Park
1775 Water Place
Atlanta, GA 30339

Crunch Gwinnett
Gwinnett Prado
2300 Pleasant Hill Road
Duluth, GA 30136

Crunch Town Center
Main Street Shopping
  Center
2600 Prado Lane
Marietta, GA 30066

Crunch Roswell
Roswell Exchange
11060 Alpharetta Highway
Roswell, GA 30076

Crunch Buckhead
3365 Piedmont Road,
Suite 1010
Atlanta, GA

Crunch Stone Mountain
Stone Mountain Square
5370 Highway 78 South
Stone Mountain, GA 30087

TOKYO

Crunch Omotesando
4-3-24 Jingumae Sibuya

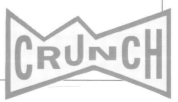

CHICAGO AND LAS VEGAS COMING SOON!